The Tao of Detox

Also by Daniel Reid

Guarding the Three Treasures
The Tao of Health, Sex & Longevity
Chi-Gung

The Tao of Detox

The Natural Way to Purify Your Body for Health and Longevity

DANIEL REID

Illustrations by
Dexter Chou

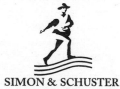

SIMON & SCHUSTER

LONDON • NEW YORK • SYDNEY • TOKYO • SINGAPORE • TORONTO • DUBLIN

A VIACOM COMPANY

First published in Great Britain by Simon & Schuster UK Ltd, 2003
A Viacom Company

1 3 5 7 9 10 8 6 4 2

Simon & Schuster UK Ltd
Africa House
64–78 Kingsway
London WC2B 6AH

www.simonsays.co.uk

Simon & Schuster Australia
Sydney

A CIP catalogue record for this book is available from the British Library

ISBN 0–7432–3210–0

Typeset by Palimpsest Book Production Limited,
Polmont, Stirlingshire
Printed and bound in Great Britain by
The Bath Press, Bath

This book is dedicated to
V.E. Irons
for getting to the bottom of the problem
and showing us the way to fix it,
and to
Marlene and Julia
for keeping his good work going.

Contents

Preface

Despite the 'wonders of modern medicine', the state of human health throughout the world today continues to erode at an alarming rate. This deterioration prevails as much in the wealthy, industrially developed parts of the world as it does in poor, underdeveloped regions. America, for example, has one of the highest per capita rates of cancer mortality on earth, and the immune deficiency syndrome known as AIDS has spread to every corner of the planet, striking the rich as well as the poor, old and young alike. Debilitating diseases and chronic degenerative conditions that only a hundred years ago rarely manifested except in the weak and elderly have today become increasingly common conditions in the young and mainstream adult sectors of the population. Chronic pain and fatigue, indigestion and insomnia, hypertension and heart failure, and all sorts of other maladies are now par for the course in the lives of men and women all over the world, degrading the quality of their lives and causing untold misery.

So what's the problem here?

The problem is toxicity, plain and simple, the same sort of toxicity that attracts flies to filth, kills fish in rivers, and lays waste to the environment, except in this case we're talking about the toxic waste that pollutes the blood and tissues of the human body. Modern Western lifestyle, particularly the highly touted 'American way of life', has spread like an oil slick across the entire sea of humanity, smothering traditional ways of life that once kept the human body in a relatively healthy state of balance. Fast food and junk food, preservatives and additives, chemically contaminated air and water, mad-dash lifestyles and indiscriminate use of drugs, both medical and recreational, have all contributed to the overall degradation of human health and the relentless pollution of the human body.

Most people today take far better care of their cars than they do their own bodies. Imagine what would happen if you indiscriminately poured petrol, diesel, kerosene, propane and a cup of sugar altogether into the petrol tank of your car. That's precisely the way most people eat today, mixing meat, bread, milk, fat, sugar and other digestively incompatible foods at the same meals and pouring them into their stomachs at the same time. And what if you never changed the motor oil, neglected to clean the filters, and let the carburettor get crusted up with soot? The result would be obvious: the fuel would burn inefficiently, producing foul-smelling toxic wastes and gases, the engine would soon begin to wheeze and splutter, vital moving parts would seize up and malfunction, and finally the whole machine would grind to a shuddering halt and need to be hauled to the nearest repair shop. All of this could be easily prevented, and expensive repair work avoided, simply by keeping the engine properly tuned, periodically changing the oil and replacing the filters, cleaning the carburettor, using the right type of fuel, and properly maintaining the vehicle on a daily basis.

Many of today's most common and deadly diseases, such as cancer, diabetes and cirrhosis of the liver, are caused not by viruses or other germs, but rather by long-term accumulation of toxins and acid wastes in the body, which create the conditions of tissue toxicity that germs require to infect the body. Similarly, most chronic degenerative conditions, such as arthritis, arterio-sclerosis and immune deficiency, are acquired primarily as a result of blood and tissue toxicity produced from things that people put into their own bodies. As these acidic toxins fester and decay in various tissues, they damage organs and glands, corrode joints and arteries, enervate the nervous system and inhibit immune response and other vital functions. This debili-tating state of tissue toxicity is almost always self-inflicted, and it cannot be corrected with pills, injections, surgery or any other 'quick-fix' medical procedures. The one and only way to counter-act self-toxification of the body is by self-detoxification, and the only one who can do that for you is the same person who allowed it to happen in the first place – you. As the saying goes, 'It's a dirty job, but someone has to do it', and in this case that someone is you.

Fortunately, there are simple ways to get the job of detox done quickly and efficiently and to repair the damage that toxicity does to vital organs and functions. However, it's entirely up to you to take the time and apply the discipline required to detoxify your system properly, and to do so on a regular basis, just the way you care for your car with periodic tune-ups and proper daily maintenance. Life is toxic by nature, and just as fire invari-ably produces smoke and ash, so the metabolic processes of life quickly begin to 'retox' your body the moment you've finished a detox programme. Therefore, the secret to enjoying a long and healthy life – and being able to 'eat, drink, and be merry' while also working, prospering and remaining fit – is to practise the discipline of periodic detox and apply the principles of 'rational retox' to your daily life.

In the Far East, where people like to work hard, play hard and enjoy every aspect of life, health and longevity have always been cultivated as the two most precious treasures of life, and they form the cornerstones upon which the enjoyment and accomplishment of everything else worth doing depends.

Regardless of how busy they became in the relentless pursuit of fame and fortune, food and sex, prosperity and pleasure, people in traditional Asian societies always took the time to relax their bodies and rest their minds, to replenish their energies and rebalance their systems, and designed their diets and other basic habits in ways that protected their health and prolonged their lives, rather than hastened their degeneration and demise. By following these basic principles, traditional Eastern cultures developed a knack for healthy living that enhances rather than diminishes the enjoyment of life's pleasures, and assists rather than interferes with the demands of hard work. The Japanese, for example, who work harder by day and play harder by night than anyone else on earth, and who live with the most intense forms of modern industrial pollution, continue to enjoy the longest average lifespan in the world, simply by continuing to follow traditional ways in their personal habits of life. What they and other East Asian cultures have learned is the ancient Chinese art of longevity by means of toxic damage control, a system known as the 'way of nurturing life' (*yang-sheng dao*). In other words, they practised the 'Tao of detox'.

The 'way of nurturing life' is a comprehensive system of self-health care that is as relevant to the human condition today as it was when first developed over 3,000 years ago in ancient China, and the life-prolonging benefits for those who practise this way of life are greater today than ever before. In *The Tao of Health, Sex & Longevity*, I introduce this system of self-purification as follows:

> The essential principle is to combat the debilitating, deathly effects of environmental poisons and self-pollution with the rejuvenating, death-defying antidote of personal hygiene and self-purification . . . The purpose of regular regimens of self-cleansing is simply to stay a few steps ahead of the inexorable process of pollution and decay. 'Aging' is not a matter of time

alone; it is the *rate* at which we permit our bodies to decay over a period of time.

Having practised these methods myself for nearly 30 years, I agree with their principles more than ever, and I wholeheartedly endorse this system as the best way to protect your health, preserve your vitality and prolong your life.

This book presents the most practical and effective methods used for thousands of years in traditional East Asian cultures to cultivate health and longevity through personal hygiene and proper daily care of the human body. The therapeutic powers of these ancient Eastern healing arts are further amplified by fusing them with modern technology and new health products, and their basic principles are more clearly illuminated by viewing them in the light of modern medical science. By selectively blending the best of East and West in self-health care, this book presents a comprehensive system for protecting health and prolonging life by means of internal cleansing, and introduces a variety of practical programmes that anyone can learn to practise within the context of one's own daily life.

However, a book can only show you the way; the will to follow it can only come from you. Hopefully, this book will inspire that wish in you.

Daniel Reid
Byron Bay, Australia
February 2002

Tissue Toxicity

In recent years, environmental pollution and the poisoning of our food, air and water supplies have become issues of major concern and hot debate throughout the world, but virtually nothing has been done to correct these problems or reverse the trend. In fact, as the population of the planet continues to multiply and the pace of industrialization continues to accelerate, the poisoning of life on earth grows more severe and widespread day by day.

Along with this radical degradation of our living environment has come an equally swift erosion in the quality of human health: cancer, AIDS, heart disease, liver infection, respiratory ailments, nervous disorders and a host of other maladies have spread like wildfire throughout the general population all over the world, ravaging lives in all segments of society. For all its highly touted surgical weaponry and massive arsenal of chemical drugs, conventional medicine has failed to defend humanity against this malignant attack. Rather than protecting people from this relentless onslaught of disease and degeneration, modern allopathic medicine simply tries to manage its symptoms with drugs and surgery, and the treatment often leads to even worse symptoms later.

What modern medicine, as well as most victims of disease today, fail to recognize is the direct correlation between external pollution of the environment and internal pollution of the human body. The simple fact is this: whatever poisons are put into the macrocosmic eco-systems of nature invariably seep into the microcosmic bio-systems of human health. External toxicity of food, air and water always cause internal toxicity of blood, tissues and cellular fluids, and these toxic conditions become the breeding ground for disease and degeneration. No drug or surgical procedure can correct this problem, because the cause is not germs, genes or congenital defects. The cause is a state of toxicity in the blood and tissues of the human body, a condition known as toxaemia. If you see a festering pile of rubbish crawling with flies and maggots, you don't blame the flies for creating the filth, and you don't try to get rid of it by poisoning the flies and maggots with chemicals. What you do is get rid of the rubbish and clean up the mess it made, in which case the flies and maggots have no place left to breed, and they disappear naturally, thereby solving the problem without waging chemical warfare against nature.

The same principle applies to human health. The only real way to cure any chronic disease or degenerative condition is to eliminate the root cause by ridding the body of the toxins that pollute the blood and tissues, attract germs and weaken resistance and immunity. That means detoxifying the internal environment of the human body, repairing the toxic damage done to vital organs, and restoring balance to all the basic vital functions. When the blood and tissues of the body have been purged of poisons, germs cannot attack, degeneration is arrested, and the body's natural healing mechanisms repair the damage and restore optimum health to the whole system. Until the world wakes up to the mortal danger which environmental pollution poses to human health and longevity, and takes effective measures to clean up the planet, human beings who wish to live long and healthy lives in this world have no choice but to take their own measures to periodically detoxify and protect the inner world of their own bodies, and to try to stay a few steps ahead of the constant retoxification process that occurs naturally in the course of daily life.

Even without environmental pollution, the human body produces internal toxins as a natural by-product of digestion and metabolism. When glucose and oxygen are burned in the cells to create energy, acid wastes and other toxic by-products such as carbon dioxide are produced. Lactic acid, for example, is a toxic waste produced in the tissues as a result of muscular exertion. When new cells grow to replace damaged cells, the old cells are dismantled and dissolved by enzymes, and this cellular debris becomes more toxic waste that must be removed from the body. In a healthy, well balanced body, all of this natural metabolic waste is automatically eliminated from the system by the excretory organs. As the eminent American physician Dr John Tilden writes in his book *Toxemia*, 'Toxin is a by-product as constant and necessary as life itself. When the organism is normal, it is produced and eliminated as fast as produced.'

A normal, healthy body will therefore naturally detoxify itself by eliminating its own self-produced toxic wastes as fast as they are produced. Toxaemia occurs, and the conditions for disease are thereby created, when toxins are retained and stored in the body due to toxic overload or impairment of the body's own natural detox and elimination functions. As Dr Tilden states, 'Without toxemia there can be no disease . . . Thus retention of metabolic toxin is the first and only cause of disease . . . One of the first things to do to get rid of any so-called disease is to get rid of toxemia, for it is this state of the blood that makes disease possible.' Dr Theodore Baroody, author of *Alkalize or Die*, agrees emphatically with this view:

> The countless names attached to illnesses do not really
> matter. What does matter is that they all come from
> the same root cause . . . too much tissue acid waste in

the body! . . . It is these tissue residues that determine sickness or health!

Retention of toxins within the body has two basic causes: one is massive toxic overload beyond natural metabolic levels due to excess exposure to unnatural environmental toxins in food, air and water; the other is impairment of normal elimination processes due to unhealthy personal habits, exhaustion and ener-vation of the nervous system caused by hyperactive modern lifestyles. In most cases, toxaemia is the net result of a combi-nation of various factors – indiscriminate eating habits and chem-ically contaminated food and water; smoking and drinking, a 'fast-lane' lifestyle of hard work and hard play; excessive stress and insufficient rest; and so forth. But regardless of the sources of toxicity, the net result is always the same – a state of toxaemia – and toxaemia is the root cause of all disease and degeneration. Therefore, the first step in curing any disease, correcting its cause, and preventing the onset of other diseases is to detoxify the whole system, just as cleaning up the rubbish is the only way to get rid of flies and maggots. After each period of intensive detox, you may then take appropriate measures to 'clean up your act' in daily life, so that retox proceeds more slowly and less severely than before. This involves changing some of your eating habits, adjusting various aspects of your lifestyle, and learning a few basic rules that govern the way your body works, such as the axiom, 'You are what you eat'.

One of the most important things to learn about how your body works, especially with regard to detox and retox, is the way the autonomic nervous system operates. All of the body's vital functions are controlled by the autonomic nervous system, which has two antagonistic branches. One is called the sympathetic branch, also known as the 'action circuit' or 'fight or flight' response ('F or F'). This is the branch that is switched on by any sort of physical exertion, hard work, excitement, sensory stimulation, emotional turmoil and any other intensive activity. When the 'F or F' action circuit is switched on, the body's entire supply of nervous energy is consumed in active response to external conditions, emotional reactions and sensory stimulation, and these functions burn up nerve energy faster than it can be produced. The result of such neuro-active depletion is a state of nervous exhaustion or enervation, which has become a chronic condition of daily life for the majority of people throughout the world today.

The other branch of the nervous system is called the parasympathetic circuit, and it is this branch that governs the immune system, controls auto-detoxification and self-cleansing responses, and regulates excretory functions. It is also known as the 'rest and relaxation' circuit ('R & R'), because the one and only way to activate this branch and allow it to function properly is to give both body and mind a period of complete rest and total relaxation. The human body was designed to function in a healthy state of balance between these two modes of nervous response: intensive bursts of activity in the sympathetic 'F or F' action circuit are supposed to be followed by periods of deep rest and physical relaxation in the parasympathetic 'R & R' healing circuit in order to allow the system to recuperate and rebalance itself. Whenever the nervous system is locked into the intensive action mode for prolonged periods of time, such as in modern urban lifestyles, immune response atrophies, cleansing and excretory functions are suppressed and toxic wastes continuously accumulate in the body, setting the stage for disease and decay. Only when the nervous system is at rest in the restorative parasympathetic mode can the body neutralize and eliminate toxins, process and excrete digestive wastes and restore itself to a balanced state of health that promotes long life.

Today, virtually everyone in the world finds themselves locked into the hyperactive, depleting, highly toxifying sympathetic branch of the autonomic nervous system, with very little time to spend in the healing, restorative parasympathetic mode. The modern lifestyle, with its 'work hard, play hard' ethic, makes little allowance for sustained periods of rest and relaxation. Over-work, over-indulgence in food and drink, over-stimulation of the senses and over-excitement of the emotions all conspire to keep the action circuit of the human nervous system switched on day and night, and this leads to a state of constant enerva-tion and toxic overload. This in turn produces conditions of chronic toxaemia, which is the root cause of most disease and degeneration. As Dr Tilden puts it, 'Toxemia is the cause of all disease, and enervation – an enervated body and mind – is the cause of toxemia.' The only solution here is to give body and mind a prolonged period of complete rest and total relaxation, thereby switching the nervous system over to the healing mode of the parasympathetic branch and allowing the entire body to cleanse and purify itself naturally, replenish its energy reserves, and restore its normal resistance to disease and degeneration.

Let's take a closer look at the basic nature of toxaemia. In a normal healthy body, the blood and most other bodily fluids should be slightly alkaline, very much like seawater, and the tissues and cells should be well oxygenated. Alkaline and oxygen are therefore the twin pillars of good health and strong immune response. Bacterial, viral and fungal infections cannot develop in tissues that are sufficiently alkalized and oxygenated, and almost all microbes and toxins are neutralized by the presence of alkaline and oxygen elements. However, when internal toxi-city exceeds the body's capacity to cleanse itself, alkaline and oxygen levels plummet, and a state of toxaemia develops. This state is characterized by two primary conditions: excess acid (acidosis) and insufficient oxygen (hypoxia).

Acidosis and hypoxia are the underlying conditions that allow bacteria, viruses, fungus and other microbes to invade and breed inside the human body. Virtually all germs that infect the human body are anaerobic, which means that they thrive in oxygen-deficient environments, such as toxic tissues. Ever since Louis Pasteur proposed his germ theory of disease, modern Western medicine has become obsessed with the simplistic view that every disease must be caused by the specific germs which appear in diseased tissues, and that the cure for any particular disease is to kill the specific germ associated with its symptoms. As a result, modern Western medicine engages in an ever escalating campaign of 'chemical warfare' against germs, fought on the battleground of the human body. This approach fails entirely to account for the fact that under precisely the same conditions of exposure, some people become infected by germs and get sick, while others do not. The difference between those who 'catch' germs and those who don't is that those who do have lower resistance than those who don't. As the famous American physician Dr Charles Mayo stated, 'We are all afraid of germs because we are all ignorant of them. Germs are outside, what we should be afraid of is lowered resistance from within.'

Viewing the situation from the rubbish and fly analogy, people whose blood and tissues are littered with accumulations of toxic debris are the ones who become most vulnerable to infection by germs, just as rubbish attracts flies. All microbes have a very narrow range of conditions in which they can survive and reproduce. The two most basic conditions that allow pathogenic microbes to colonize human tissues are excess acidity and insufficient oxygen. Any wine or beer maker can testify to the fact that the bacteria they use to ferment their products require an acid medium of very specific degree, without exposure to oxygen, in order to function. On his deathbed, Pasteur himself finally recanted his germ theory by admitting that 'the terrain is everything'. Without the specific preconditions of acidosis and hypoxia, germs simply cannot survive in the 'terrain' of human tissues, just as flies cannot breed in the terrain of a sanitary environment. What this means is that the presence of germs in the blood is not the root cause of any disease, but rather a *symptom* of toxaemia.

Toxaemia provides the breeding ground for germs and thereby becomes the root cause of all disease.

The implications of this fact find their greatest significance in the understanding and treatment of cancer. In 1931, Dr Otto Warburg received the Nobel Prize for medicine for his discovery that *all* forms of cancer, without exception, are characterized by two basic conditions: acidosis and hypoxia. Like germs, cancer cells flourish only in acidic, anaerobic environments, in which they reproduce as rapidly as fermenting bacteria. This discovery clearly indicates that the best way to cure and prevent cancer is to alkalize and oxygenate the blood and tissues, thereby eliminating the conditions in which cancer cells thrive. However, modern medicine has totally ignored Dr Warburg's work, and has chosen instead to attack cancer the same way it attacks germs: poisoning it with toxic chemical drugs, burning it with radiation therapy and cutting it out with radical surgery. None of these conventional cancer treatments provides a real cure for the underlying cause of cancer; in fact, they further aggravate the root cause by strongly elevating the levels of tissue toxicity, while at the same time severely inhibiting the body's own natural cleansing and healing responses.

A hundred years ago, less than one in a thousand people died of cancer. In the UK today, one in three people will be diagnosed with cancer in their lifetime, and one in every four will die. Having clearly lost the 'war on cancer' long ago, modern medicine nevertheless stubbornly continues to ignore its root causes and now claims that people get cancer due to a 'genetic predisposition' to it, as though cancer were an inherited trait, like freckles and blue eyes. This is nonsense. While 5–10 per cent of cancer cases may be linked in some way to faulty genes, if most cancers were genetically determined, as some doctors now claim, then a hundred years ago the incidence of cancer should have been about the same as it is today, rather than 250 times lower. Mainstream medicine has taken the wrong track on cancer treatment but refuses to admit it because cancer therapy has become one of the most profitable branches of the modern medical industry. Meanwhile, these conventional therapies continue to make matters much worse for cancer patients by increasing the underlying state of toxaemia that lies at the root cause of all cancer.

The fact is that 80–90 per cent of all cancer cases can be traced back to basic environmental factors, of which diet is by far the most important. Toxins assimilated from external sources accumulate and fester inside the body, causing internal toxicity of blood and tissues and producing the conditions of acidosis and anaerobia upon which cancer feeds. The answer to cancer is to clean up the cumulative tissue toxicity that allows cancer to develop in the first place, and to stop using the human body as a dumping ground for all the toxic waste that enters the system with food, water, air, smoke, drugs and other external sources. There's no way to totally avoid toxic contamination these days, but you can certainly reduce your risk by making some basic changes in your diet and lifestyle and taking a few simple preventive measures, and you can certainly protect yourself from cancer, heart disease and other life-threatening ailments by periodically flushing the poisons that cause them out of your system, rather than letting them accumulate to critical levels.

If cancer is detected early enough, before it causes irreversible damage to vital organs, it can usually be treated and cured by a combination of various detoxification methods, such as fasting and colonic irrigation, raw juice and detox diet therapy, herbal and nutritional supplements, alkalization and oxygenation of blood and tissues, and other holistic methods, without the need for debilitating toxic treatments such as chemotherapy, radiation and radical surgery. However, if a doctor tells a patient that cancer can be cured by means of blood and tissue detox, and offers to provide such a cure, they are likely to be prosecuted. It is not 'politically correct' these days for doctors to discuss the real causes of cancer, nor to provide real cures that work, because

the profits of powerful pharmaceutical cartels and other branches
of the modern medical industry are threatened by the truth
regarding the real causes and cures for disease. It's therefore up
to each of us to discover the truth ourselves, and act on it by
taking effective preventive measures to protect our health and
prolong our lives in a world that grows progressively more toxic
and 'user-unfriendly'.

Cancer is the final, fatal stage of tissue toxicity, but it takes a
long time to develop, and long before it does, chronic toxaemia
takes its toll on human health in many other ways, making life
miserable for millions of people who don't realize that the root
cause of their misery is their own blood and tissue toxicity. In
addition to providing fertile ground for infection by germs,
toxaemia also damages vital organs and impairs immune
response, causing a wide range of degenerative ailments that
grow steadily worse for as long as the state of toxicity continues.
Listed below are some of the most common symptoms associated with blood acidosis and tissue toxicity:

heartburn	loss of hair
allergies	arthritis
headaches	foul body odour
festering sores	frequent colds
fungal infections	vaginitis
gastritis	depression
psoriasis	excess mucus
sinusitus	hyperactivity and anxiety
fatigue	all forms of cancer

While a variety of secondary factors such as malnutrition and
harmful habits may also be contributing causes in these conditions, the root cause always remains the same – toxaemia. Even
if the secondary factors are eliminated, the condition will
continue to manifest until the internal toxicity that allowed it to

develop in the first place is neutralized and the toxins are eliminated from the system.

The one and only solution to pollution is purification. In the case of internal pollution of the human body, and the state of chronic toxaemia that it causes, that means periodic purification of the bloodstream and complete detoxification of the bodily tissues. Unless you choose to reside in a remote mountain cave and live on nothing but wild fruit and spring water, there is no way to avoid the accumulation of toxic residues in your body. As long as the amount of toxin does not exceed the capacity of your immune and excretory systems to eliminate it, health and vitality are easily maintained, but sooner or later the toxic overload of daily life exceeds your body's ability to properly cleanse itself of it, and that's when toxaemia develops and disease and degeneration begin. The worst mistake of all is to start using pharmaceutical drugs and surgical procedures to temporarily ease the symptomic discomfort and inconvenience of the chronic diseases and degenerative conditions caused by toxaemia, because that approach only makes the problem worse by increasing blood and tissue toxicity, while weakening immune response and other vital functions. The only effective way to deal with toxaemia is to 'clean up your act' with a regular programme of detox and a rational approach to retox. This means periodically purging the blood and tissues of accumulated toxic residues, then reforming the personal lifestyle habits that contribute most to acidosis and tissue toxicity.

In order for any detox programme to be effective, you must take *at least* three days of complete rest and total relaxation. Seven days is even better, because it takes exactly seven days of complete rest and clean living to purify the bloodstream and cleanse the internal organs. Only a prolonged period of 'R&R' will allow the autonomic nervous system to switch over to the restorative parasympathetic circuit long enough to give the body a chance to completely cleanse and rebalance itself, while giving the over-worked, over-stimulated sympathetic action circuit a long overdue rest. Remember: effective detoxification and repair of the body can only take place when the mind is at rest and the nervous system is operating in the healing mode of the parasympathetic branch. There is no way you can do it simply by eating the right foods and taking the right supplements, while still remaining locked into the hectic activities of ordinary daily life. So unless you're willing to retreat from daily life for a while and take the time to do it properly, there's not much point in trying to detox at all.

Besides purging the blood and tissues of toxic residues, a period of detox also provides other essential long-term benefits for health and longevity. One of those benefits is to cleanse and rejuvenate the entire excretory system – clearing clogged bowels and congested lungs, cleaning dirty lymph and blemished skin, and flushing out dirty kidneys and bladder. The more toxic you become, the less efficiently your excretory organs work, and if extreme toxaemia continues for too long, serious organic damage to the excretory organs can occur. Another benefit of periodic detox is restoration of maximum immunity and resistance, which depends on adequate alkalization and oxygenation of the blood and cellular fluids. Bacteria and other germs simply cannot survive in a body that is sufficiently alkaline and oxygenated. Even a microbe as aggressive as anthrax can only infect a person whose body is already in a toxic state of acidosis and anaerobia, and this explains why, under precisely the same degree of exposure, some people 'catch' it and others do not. These days, with all the hazardous chemicals and microbes that contaminate our living environment, spending three to seven days once or twice a year doing a serious detox programme certainly seems worth the investment of time and effort.

The basic problem of toxaemia and the solution of detox are summarized in the schematic diagram opposite:

The Problem:	*The Solution:*
stress (environmental pollution; daily life)	rest (peace and quiet; clean living)
↓	↓
strain	relaxation
↓	↓
(physical/mental/emotional, overwork, exhaustion, worry)	(physical/mental/emotional, tranquility, comfort, support)
↓	↓
enervation (overdrive in sympathetic mode)	regeneration (rest in parasympathetic mode, replenish energy, restore vital functions)
↓	↓
inefficient elimination (bowels, lungs, kidneys, skin)	swift and effecient elimination (bowels, lungs, kidneys, skin)
↓	↓
retention of toxic wastes	elimination of toxic wastes
↓	↓
toxaemia (acidosis and anaerobia)	purification (alkalization and oxygenation)
↓	↓
acute disease, chronic degenerative conditions, cancer	immunity and resistance, health and longevity

The importance of a sustained period of rest and relaxation as an absolute prerequisite for any detox programme to be effective cannot be over-emphasized, especially in today's fast-paced, high-stress world, where resting quietly and doing nothing is regarded as a 'waste of time'. As Dr Tilden notes, 'The present day strenuousness causes enervation which checks elimination, and the retained toxins bring on toxemia . . . Rest from habits that enervate is the only way to put nature in line for healing. Sleep and rest of body and mind are necessary to keep a sufficient supply of energy. Few people in active life rest enough.' This means taking a break not only from hard work and hard play, but also from worry, anger and all other forms of emotional excitement and strong sensory stimulation, all of which enervate the nervous system, inhibit immune response and impede efficient elimination of toxins from the body.

If you cannot find sufficient peace and quiet to detox at home, or if you lack the discipline to conduct your own detox programme, the best solution is to check into a quiet, comfortable spa or health resort that has the facilities required to support an effective programme of detoxification and rejuvenation. Such resorts are becoming increasingly popular throughout the world, providing a wide range of facilities and services that not only expedite fast, efficient detoxification, but also make the entire process a lot more pleasant. Look for places located in tranquil settings next to the sea or up in the mountains, preferably those which offer facilities such as therapeutic massage, steam rooms, whirlpool baths, hot springs, raw juice bars and other restorative health regimens. Instead of always taking action holidays that leave you more exhausted and toxic than when you started, try taking a relaxing health holiday for a change, one that leaves you feeling thoroughly rested, totally refreshed and completely rejuvenated. You'll be amazed how much better you feel and how much better your body functions after allowing your system to drain out all its toxic residues, eliminate acid wastes and restore natural balance in the blood and tissues. In the following chapters, we'll discuss the best ways to accomplish this.

PART 1

Detox

CHAPTER 1

Basic Protocols of Detox

Pollution is a basic fact of life, and no one is immune to it. Although the human body is designed to cleanse itself naturally of the normal waste products of digestion and metabolism, it is clearly not equipped to deal with the additional toxic overload from chemical preservatives and pesticides, pharmaceutical drugs and artificial foods, and other sources of internal toxicity that have become common in modern lifestyles. This internal pollution is the major cause of disease, degeneration and a fore-shortened lifespan.

The most fundamental principle in Traditional Chinese Medicine (TCM) is the universal law of polarity known as the 'great principle of yin and yang'. In *The Yellow Emperor's Classic of Internal Medicine*, an important Chinese medical text written over two thousand years ago, it states, 'If it's hot [yang], cool it down [yin]. If it's empty [yin], fill it up [yang].' All traditional Chinese medical practices are based upon this principle of dynamic polarity. Extending it to the problem of blood and tissue toxicity, we could say, 'If it's polluted [yang], purify it [yin]. If it's acidic [yang], alkalize it [yin].'

Unfortunately, like so many other dichotomies in life, the purification process is not nearly as much fun, nor as easy, as the pollution process, and therefore most people tend to overlook the importance of self-detoxification, or pretend that it's not necessary. In fact, however, purification of polluted blood and tissues is absolutely necessary in order to preserve health and prolong life, particularly in the hazardous environmental conditions that prevail throughout the world today. Periodic detoxification is the best way to purge the body of both its own natural toxins as well as the unnatural and far more dangerous toxins assimilated from external sources. By taking measures to purify your blood and tissues on a regular basis, you prevent toxaemia and protect yourself from its debilitating effects, particularly the acidosis and hypoxia which make tissues vulnerable to cancer. Since acidosis and hypoxia are the primary conditions of imbalance that permit germs to breed, tissues to degenerate and cancer to develop, periodic detox is probably the single most effective preventive measure you can take to protect your life from the entire spectrum of disease and degenerative conditions. Detox is also the best cure for most of these conditions.

Flushing out acids

The first and foremost strategy in any detox programme is to flush acid residues out of the blood, lymph and other bodily fluids, which should be slightly alkaline. Almost all toxins in the body take the form of acids, and these acids must therefore be neutralized and flushed out of the system in order to restore normal alkaline balance to the blood and other bodily fluids. In TCM, the blood, lymph, bile and other essential fluids of the body are collectively referred to as *jing-yi* ('vital fluids'), and the condition of a person's *jing-yi*, particularly the bloodstream, is regarded as a primary determining factor in human health and disease.

The late V. E. Irons, one of the Western world's leading authorities on therapeutic detoxification for health and longevity, agrees with the traditional Chinese view regarding the condition of the bloodstream as a critical indicator of health and disease. As Irons

puts it, 'Every cell in the body is served by the blood. It nourishes the cell, replaces worn out parts, and carries away waste
products.' Obviously, a polluted bloodstream carries little nourishment and is already so saturated with wastes that it cannot
properly fulfill its function of carrying away cellular wastes.

The same goes for the lymphatic system. There are 600–700
lymph glands in the body, and there is about three times more
fluid volume of lymph than there is blood in the human body.
One of the primary functions of the lymph is to clean acid wastes
from the blood and tissues, but if the lymph itself is polluted
with acid wastes, then it cannot properly perform these cleansing
functions. Acids interfere with the free flow of lymph within the
lymphatic channels, thereby further inhibiting its capacity to
cleanse the blood and tissues.

Regardless of what type of detox programme you choose, you
must always remember to drink at least 2–3 litres per day of
pure, preferably alkaline water, in order to neutralize, dilute and
flush away the large amounts of acids and other toxic wastes
which the detox process releases from tissues throughout the
body. The human body is composed of over 70 per cent water.
By saturating the system daily with abundant quantities of pure
alkaline water, pollutants are continuously flushed from the
blood and tissues and eliminated through the kidneys, bowels
and skin. As a result, all bodily tissues are 'washed' and all vital
fluids are replenished with fresh water. This is equivalent to
changing the dirty motor oil in your car, as well as the battery,
brake and transmission fluids. The whole mechanism operates
more efficiently and produces less toxic waste, when dirty fluids
are replaced with clean.

Restoring proper pH balance

The corollary protocol to flushing out acids is to restore proper
pH balance in the blood and tissues. 'pH' is a standard measure

of acid/alkaline balance, calibrated on a scale of 1 (extremely acid) to 14 (extremely alkaline), with 7 as neutral. Each of our vital bodily fluids has a very specific pH level at which it functions best. Except for stomach fluids and a few others, most of our vital fluids and tissues should be slightly alkaline. Blood, for example, has a slightly alkaline pH value of 7.3 to 7.4, exactly the same as seawater. If blood pH drops below 7.1 or rises above 7.5, severe symptoms of imbalance will manifest immediately, and if pH is not quickly restored to proper balance, death follows swiftly.

Almost all forms of internal toxicity cause a state of acidosis in the body. In turn, excessive levels of acid residues in the blood and tissues suppress immune response, interfere with normal metabolism, inhibit digestion and assimilation, promote fungal and bacterial infections, and cause all sorts of other biological malfunctions and ill health. To give you an idea of how important pH balance is throughout the human system, here are some of the ways your vital organs depend upon proper pH balance to function correctly:

Heart
The human heart pumps about 130 litres of blood per hour. If the blood is saturated with acid wastes, the acids can do serious damage to heart tissue as the blood passes through it, gradually causing deterioration of the heart muscle. Moreover, normal heartbeat rhythms are dependent on an alkaline environment and are therefore adversely affected by excess acid wastes in the bloodstream. And since acid wastes drastically reduce the blood's capacity to carry oxygen, the heart does not receive sufficient oxygen supplies from blood that's saturated with acids.

Lungs
One way that the body can self-regulate pH balance in the blood is by controlling the oxygen level through correct breathing. By

maximizing the exchange of gases in the lungs, proper diaphragmatic breathing saturates the bloodstream with fresh supplies of oxygen, while purging it of carbon dioxide. Oxygen supports an alkaline environment in the blood and tissues, while carbon dioxide contributes to acidosis. If you permit your blood to become overloaded with acid wastes, it cannot absorb and carry sufficient oxygen from the lungs to sustain an alkaline blood and tissue pH, resulting instead in a state of chronic hypoxia (oxygen deficiency) and its twin condition acidosis, in every tissue and cell in the body. This in turn paves the way for germs and tumours to develop.

Liver

One of the liver's main jobs is to filter toxic wastes from the bloodstream. Another task is to produce many of the alkaline enzymes upon which immune response and other vital functions depend. If the blood is constantly polluted by excess acid residues from wrong eating habits, alcohol and drugs, stress hormones and other acid-forming factors, the liver eventually gets overloaded with acid wastes and becomes deeply congested with toxic debris. This is turn impairs its ability to filter acids from the bloodstream, so instead the body starts depositing excess acid wastes in the joints and other solid tissues, causing arthritis and tissue toxicity throughout the body.

Kidneys

The kidneys also help to filter acid wastes from the bloodstream, processing about one litre of blood per minute. This is turn helps keep blood pH at its proper alkaline level. Excessive acid waste in the blood due to improper diet, pharmaceutical drugs and other lifestyle factors can severely corrode the delicate tissues in which blood filters through the kidneys. It can also cause the formation of kidney stones and inflammation of the bladder and urinary tract.

maximizing the exchange of gases in the lungs, proper diaphragmatic breathing saturates the bloodstream with fresh supplies of oxygen, while purging it of carbon dioxide. Oxygen supports an alkaline environment in the blood and tissues, while carbon dioxide contributes to acidosis. If you permit your blood to become overloaded with acid wastes, it cannot absorb and carry sufficient oxygen from the lungs to sustain an alkaline blood and tissue pH, resulting instead in a state of chronic hypoxia (oxygen deficiency) and its twin condition acidosis, in every tissue and cell in the body. This in turn paves the way for germs and tumours to develop.

Liver
One of the liver's main jobs is to filter toxic wastes from the bloodstream. Another task is to produce many of the alkaline enzymes upon which immune response and other vital functions depend. If the blood is constantly polluted by excess acid residues from wrong eating habits, alcohol and drugs, stress hormones and other acid-forming factors, the liver eventually gets overloaded with acid wastes and becomes deeply congested with toxic debris. This is turn impairs its ability to filter acids from the bloodstream, so instead the body starts depositing excess acid wastes in the joints and other solid tissues, causing arthritis and tissue toxicity throughout the body.

Kidneys
The kidneys also help to filter acid wastes from the bloodstream, processing about one litre of blood per minute. This is turn helps keep blood pH at its proper alkaline level. Excessive acid waste in the blood due to improper diet, pharmaceutical drugs and other lifestyle factors can severely corrode the delicate tissues in which blood filters through the kidneys. It can also cause the formation of kidney stones and inflammation of the bladder and urinary tract.

way, from unpolluted seashores, and dried naturally by wind and sun.

Oxygenation is the other major method of quickly restoring pH balance in the blood, and the best way to utilize this method is simply by learning to breathe properly, using the diaphragm rather than the upper chest to drive the breath. Sufficient oxygenation is an essential factor for maintaining an adequately alkaline environment in the blood and tissues. Conversely, progressive acidosis of blood and tissues is always associated with insufficient oxygenation, and therefore increasing oxygen supplies to the blood and tissues is an antidote to acidosis. In addition to learning how to breathe correctly and practising deep breathing exercises, you can also oxygenate your blood and tissues by taking various types of oxygen supplements, such as water oxygenated with ozone, a few drops of hydrogen peroxide in a glass of water, deuterium sulphate ('ESF'), ionized alkaline micro-cluster water (microwater), and others. We'll take a closer look at some of these products in the next chapter.

Dredging the drains

During any detox programme, the organs of elimination must work overtime to process and excrete all the accumulated toxic wastes that are loosened and released from organs and tissues throughout the body. Since the organs of elimination are already overworked from dealing with environmental pollution and wrong eating habits, the extra load of toxins that are suddenly released into the bloodstream, bowels, kidneys and skin by the detox process can put a very heavy strain on the excretory organs. It is therefore important to give your excretory systems all the supplemental support you can during detox, to ensure maximum efficiency in elimination, with minimum toxic stress to the organs.

There are four main 'drains' in the body through which toxic waste products are excreted from the system: the skin, the b the kidneys and bladder, and the colon. As your blood and tissues grow progressively more toxic during the course of daily life, these drains get clogged with toxic residues, dry mucus, dead microbes and other 'bio-waste'. In the case of the colon, the situation is very similar to what happens to the drain in your kitchen sink: layer upon layer of grease, partially decayed food and other debris adhere to the pipe, gradually reducing the size of the passage through which waste water flows. And since this sticky layer of waste is full of microbes and toxins, it pollutes the bloodstream by osmosis through the colon wall, allowing the poisons to circulate throughout the body.

There are a number of ways to facilitate the drainage of toxic wastes through the four organs of elimination, and to protect them from damage during the detox process, and these will be discussed in detail in the following chapters. Briefly, here are some of the primary support protocols for each of the main drains during detox:

Skin

An enormous amount of toxic waste passes through the skin, especially in hot weather, when the pores remain open day and night. During detox, toxic residues become very concentrated in perspiration, and they can damage the skin as they pass through for excretion. Strong, foul body odour and clammy sweat are additional manifestations of heavy toxicity in perspiration during detox. Damage to skin may be prevented, as well as relieved and repaired, by soaking daily in hot baths with sea salt or Epsom salts, plus some essential oils that helps draw toxic wastes swiftly out through the pores. Another effective method of facilitating skin detox is the traditional Thai herbal steambath, which draws toxins out through the skin while also soothing skin tissue with healing herbal essences. If you're doing your detox programme by the sea, daily plunges in the ocean also provide cleansing support for the skin.

Lungs

The lungs excrete carbon dioxide and other volatile gaseous wastes from the blood, while absorbing oxygen, negative ions and other elements from the air and transferring them into the bloodstream. When the blood is highly toxic, such as during detox programmes, its capacity to carry oxygen is severely reduced, and this in turn leads to a state of hypoxia throughout the system. The anaerobic state produced by hypoxia supports an acid environment, thereby creating the conditions for disease and degeneration. Therefore, learning deep breathing exercises and practising them daily is highly recommended during any detox programme. Proper breathing oxygenates the blood and tissues, thereby helping to eliminate acidosis, while also facilitating rapid excretion of carbon dioxide and other gaseous wastes which contribute to acidosis. Thai herbal steam baths are also a very effective lung support therapy during detox: the soothing herbal essences in the steam bathe the delicate lung tissues in healing vapours with every breath, while drawing toxic residues out of the lungs. It's also a good idea to keep a negative ion generator in your room to help the lungs function smoothly and support the detox process during sleep.

Kidneys and bladder

Some of the body's most toxic wastes pass through the kidneys, which filter them from the blood and excrete them through the bladder as urine. When these wastes are highly acidic, they can damage the sensitive kidney tissues through which they filter and can also form painful kidney stones. It's therefore advisable to drink lots of herbal teas during detox, especially those with diuretic and kidney cleansing properties, in order to facilitate rapid excretion and protect the kidneys from toxic damage. Another important measure to protect the kidneys and promote swift elimination is to drink 2–3 litres of pure alkaline water daily, preferably ionized micro-clustered water. This water dilutes the concentration of toxins in the blood and kidneys, neutralizes acidity and flushes poisons quickly out of the system.

Colon

Of all the excretory organs, the colon is the most abused and overloaded these days. Believe it or not, the average Western male today carries about 5–6 kg of dense, rubbery, mucoid material – a thick toxic sludge – imbedded in his bowels, and none of it is ordinary faeces. It's the sort of deeply impacted slime that you find in the drainpipe of a clogged kitchen sink. During a detox programme, it's a very good idea to eliminate as much of this toxic lining as possible from the bowels, and to accomplish that you should take ground psyllium seed shaken in water at least twice daily, and drink plenty of extra water. The psyllium and the water gel up to form a fibrous bolus that sweeps through your bowels like a broom, loosening and eliminating mounds of impacted wastes from the walls of the bowels. For even more dramatic results and a complete cleansing of the entire colon, a series of colonic irrigations is recommended, especially during the first few days of a detox programme. In addition to cleansing the colon and eliminating a major source of toxins to the bloodstream, colonic irrigation triggers a strong detox response in the liver, and a major cleansing reaction throughout the body. It's impossible to describe in words the sheer volume and incredibly foul appearance of the putrid mucoid wastes that come tumbling out of the body with a series of colonic irrigations, after festering in the bowels for years and years. It's definitely a case of 'seeing is believing', and anyone who's ever done it can testify how good it feels to dump all that bad rubbish from their bodies.

If you really wish to 'start at the bottom' in a progressive programme to completely detoxify and regenerate your whole system, then you should definitely begin with a series of colonic irrigations to dredge your bowels of all the putrefied, partially digested debris and toxic residues that have accumulated inside over the years. This is best done in conjunction with a 3–7 day water or juice fast. Until you do this, regardless of how well you cleanse your blood and tissues by other means, the sludge in your bowels will continuously seep toxins right back into your bloodstream, and virtually everyone today has this problem. Even a hundred years ago, the famous American naturopath Dr Harvey Kellogg, who invented the corn flake and was portrayed in the novel and film *Road to Wellville*, noted, 'Of the 22,000 operations that I have personally performed, I have never found a normal colon.' V. E. Irons, who devoted his long life to promoting colon health, remarked, 'About the only place you see a normal healthy colon today is in an anatomy book!'

It's rather pointless to embark on a major new dietary programme and spend a lot of money on expensive nutritional and herbal supplements if your bowels are impacted with toxic wastes from years of pollutants and wrong eating habits. Not only does this thick slimy lining constantly secrete toxins into the bloodstream through the bowel walls, in the small intestine it blocks the assimilation of nutrients and herbal essences into the bloodstream. As Dr Norman Walker, who lived to the age of 116 by practising what he preached, states in his book *Colon Health: The Key to a Vibrant Life*:

> The elimination of undigested food and other waste products is equally important as the proper digestion and assimilation of food . . . . The very best diets can be no better than the very worst if the sewage system of the colon is clogged with a collection of waste and corruption.

Those who've done colonic irrigations always remark on how much better they feel afterwards, and how colonics often eliminate chronic conditions that defied all other treatments. Nothing facilitates internal cleansing and accelerates the detox process as effectively as colonic irrigation. If you're still a 'colonic virgin' and you really wish to know how it feels to unclog your bowels and wash them 'squeaky clean', you should gird your loins and take the plunge as the first big step on your own 'Road to Wellville'.

'Moving water, active hinges'

An ancient Chinese text on human health states, 'Moving water never stagnates; active hinges never rust.' That means if you exercise gently every day, to keep your blood, lymph and other vital bodily fluids flowing freely, and to keep your joints and other moving parts active, then your bodily fluids won't stagnate and become toxic, and your joints won't 'rust' with arthritis and stiffness. Regular, rhythmic body movements are particularly important for moving the lymph, because, unlike blood, which is pumped by the heart, lymph flow depends entirely on gravity and body movement for mobility. Since the lymph must work even harder than usual to cleanse the blood and tissues during a detox programme, it's important to help keep lymph flowing freely with daily exercise.

The type of exercise required during detox is very different from strenuous sports activities such as tennis, football, jogging and weight lifting. Western field sports and other forms of 'hard' style exercise produce lactic acid in the tissues and carbon dioxide in the bloodstream as metabolic by-products of muscular exertion, and this contributes to acidosis, which is always counterproductive to detox. One of the primary purposes of any detox programme is to eliminate acids and alkalize the system. Hard style exercise also keeps the autonomic nervous system locked into the 'fight or flight' sympathetic branch, which switches off self-cleansing and healing responses, and causes muscular tension and tightness in the joints and tendons, which interfere with the state of complete physical relaxation required for detox to proceed.

Instead of hard exercise, one should practise traditional Asian 'soft' style exercises, such as yoga, Tai Chi and *chi gung*, on a daily basis throughout the duration of any detox programme. Soft style exercise has entirely different effects on the body than hard style. The soft, slow, smooth movements of these exercises gently pump the lymph through the system, while also assisting the free circulation of blood, without causing any muscular tension and without saturating the tissues with lactic acid or overloading the blood with carbon dioxide. These gentle body movements also help dissolve and eliminate crystalline acid deposits in the joints and keep the entire skeletal structure loose and limber.

Soft style exercises should always be practised in conjunction with slow, deep, rhythmic breathing that fully engages the diaphragm. The combination of slow stretching and loosening manoeuvres with deep diaphragmatic breathing drives blood and lymph through the body like a strong pump, facilitating rapid drainage of toxins from the tissues and swift delivery of wastes to the eliminatory organs. Deep breathing greatly enhances oxygenation of the blood and tissues, which helps neutralize acidosis and maintains a healthy alkaline environment inside the body. When breathing properly, the diaphragm descends deeply into the abdominal cavity, providing an invigorating massage to the internal organs and glands. Diaphragmatic breathing gently squeezes the internal organs like a sponge on inhalation, draining out stale blood, then releases the pressure on exhalation, drawing freshly oxygenated blood into the organs. This deep diaphragmatic pressure on the internal organs and glands accelerates the detox process and extends it into the deepest, densest tissues of the body.

Most importantly, deep breathing, especially when performed in conjunction with slow rhythmic body movements, immediately produces the state of physical and mental relaxation required to switch the autonomic nervous system into the healing, restorative mode of the parasympathetic branch. Detoxification and healing can *only* proceed when the nervous system is operating in the parasympathetic circuit, and one of the primary functions of all traditional Asian soft style exercises is to activate the body's innate self-cleansing and healing mechanisms by switching the nervous system into the calm parasympathetic mode. That's what this style of exercise is designed to do, and that's why it plays such an important role in traditional Asian health and healing systems.

Pollution and purification

Pollution and purification are natural cycles of life. Like birth and death, growth and decay, and all the seasonal cycles of nature, pollution and purification follow their own natural rhythms of yin and yang phases (Fig. 1). The human body has its own built-in purification cycles to deal with the natural pollution produced by digestion, respiration and metabolism, but the

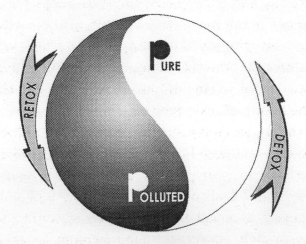

Fig. 1 **The natural cycle of pollution and purification**

system is clearly not designed to handle the enormous overload of artificial pollutants in modern life. People now living on this planet assimilate more hazardous toxins in a single day than they did in an entire lifetime only a few hundred years ago. The only way to deal with this toxic overload and prevent it from ruining your health and shortening your life is to assist your body's natural self-cleansing mechanisms with periodic detox programmes and adjustments in daily lifestyle, such as those introduced in this book, so that purification always remains a few steps ahead of pollution.

It should be noted that the programmes described in this book are designed to rid the body of the sort of blood and tissue toxicity that most people today develop in the course of daily life from such sources as poor dietary habits, environmental pollution, chemical additives in food, water, cosmetics and other household products, as well as moderate occasional use of alcohol and drugs. They are not, however, designed to treat withdrawal from long-term addiction to alcohol and drugs, which usually requires additional special support for the central nervous system. The only exception is when Neuro-Electric Therapy (NET) is used as the primary mode of withdrawal from alcohol or drug addiction, as described in Chapter 9, in which case the other detox methods presented in this book may be very effectively employed to support the drug withdrawal process. After withdrawal is complete, these programmes may be continued as a means of purifying the bloodstream and purging the tissues of toxic drug residues, and to repair damage to the internal organs and restore functional balance to the whole system, so that a normal healthy lifestyle may be resumed.

Whether you do your periodic detox work at home or at a health resort, make absolutely certain that you will not be disturbed, upset, annoyed or interrupted from start to finish. The importance of giving body and mind a complete rest and total relaxation throughout the detox process cannot be overstated, which is why it's repeated so often in this book. You must set aside a period of at least 3–7 days of complete peace and privacy, and you must remain, as much as possible, in a calm quiet state the entire time. It won't work if you relax and do your detox regimens by day, then go out drinking and carousing at night, or if you work hard all day, then come home and try to detox at night. It's also a good idea to avoid watching violent films, listening to loud music, dealing with annoying people, or doing anything else that might excite your mind or stir up your emotions during detox. The moment you get excited or upset, your autonomic nervous system snaps back into the 'F or F' action circuit, pumping stress hormones into the bloodstream and grinding the entire detox process to a halt.

There are many different ways to facilitate the detox process – hydration and hydrotherapy, diet and supplements, massage and exercise – but none of them will work properly for you unless you slow down, calm down and cool down long enough to allow your own natural healing responses a chance to work in complete harmony with these various supplemental programmes. Half the battle is simply giving yourself that prolonged period of complete, uninterrupted rest and relaxation: the parasympathetic branch of your nervous system and the built-in healing responses that it governs will do the rest for you.

Back in the late 1960s, the hippy generation advised us all to 'turn on, tune in, and drop out'. Today, we would all be a lot better advised to 'turn off' our normal daily habits and activities for a few days, to 'tune out' the rest of the world for awhile, and 'drop in' for a spell at the nearest spa or health resort, to clean out, tune up and rebalance our overworked, overplayed systems. Many adults today can't even remember what it is like to feel naturally good from the inside, so they seek a semblance of the sensation from the outside by indulging in alcohol and drugs, food and sex, money and power, all of which continuously enervate and weaken the system and end up making them feel even worse. Very few people halt their activities and retreat from the world for even as little as 24 hours, much less the 3–7 days required for proper detox. For such people, a period of detox and self-cleansing usually comes as a very enlightening experience, on many levels, and no one who's done it properly has ever regretted the time, effort or expense it requires. Indeed, detox may some day become the new 'drugless drug' of the 21st century, both for its potent therapeutic healing benefits as well as for the 'natural high' of well being and good feeling it bestows.

CHAPTER 2

Water: Hydration and Hydrotherapy

Water is the universal solvent. It is also the quintessential symbol of the Tao in Chinese philosophy. As Lao Tze states in the *Tao Teh Ching*, 'Nothing is more yielding than water / but when it attacks things hard and resistant / there is not one of them that can prevail.' With sufficient time and exposure, water can dissolve almost any toxin, hold it in solution and deliver it elsewhere for elimination. Like city sewer and industrial waste disposal systems, water is the medium required to flush waste products out of the body. Therefore, when you're detoxifying your body, you must drink extra quantities of pure alkaline water in order to dissolve, neutralize and wash away all the toxins and acid wastes that the detox process releases into the bloodstream from the tissues.

Water is also the element that extracts nutrients from food, transports them into the bloodstream and delivers them in solution into the cells for metabolism. Over 70 per cent of the human body consists of water; 90 per cent of the blood and 85 per cent of the brain are water; even the bones contain 30 per cent water. Water is thus required for the nourishment and replenishment of vital fluids, as well as for detoxifying the blood and tissues and eliminating wastes. In order to do this, good quality water must be consumed daily in sufficient quantities to perform both of these essential functions properly.

Water has a unique capacity to carry energy and information, and it may be very precisely 'programmed' to function as a potent and highly efficient tool for cleansing and healing the body. By using such diverse methods as electrolysis and magnetic fields, light and sound, oxygen and herbal essences, water may be energized and imprinted with specific information patterns to give it potent therapeutic cleansing and healing properties.

Today there are a number of effective methods, both traditional and modern technological, that anyone can utilize to specially programme water to enhance its detoxifying and purifying properties, and to improve its capacity to hydrate tissues and deliver nutrients and medicinal herbal essences into the cells. Water may be therapeutically programmed for internal as well as external use, and both applications are highly beneficial to any detox programme.

Internal uses: hydration

Chronic dehydration has become a common condition throughout the world today. It is estimated that about 75 per cent of the American population lives in a state of chronic dehydration. Levels in other industrialized countries are likely to be similar. This causes the body's natural thirst response, which is supposed to signal the body to drink water when thirsty, to be mistaken instead for hunger, prompting frequent snack binges that lead to food addictions and obesity. In a study conducted at the University of Washington, it was shown that one glass of water effectively shut off the 'midnight munchie' syndrome in 100 per cent of the dieters tested.

Dehydration produces a state of chronic toxaemia and is one of the primary causes of daytime fatigue, sluggish metabolism, depression and inability to concentrate. It also a major contributing factor in cancer. Several studies have demonstrated that by drinking five glasses of pure water per day, the average person may reduce his or her risk of colon cancer by 45 per cent, breast cancer by 80 per cent and bladder cancer by 50 per cent. Other research indicates that drinking up to eight glasses of water daily significantly relieves chronic pain in the back and joints.

Dehydration is often the hidden cause in cases of chronic pain, including headaches, and in chronic fatigue. Dehydration dries the blood and other bodily fluids, causing cells to shrink and retain their toxic wastes. When cells are properly hydrated, they expand and become active, spontaneously cleansing themselves of toxic wastes. All bodily tissues are wrapped in envelopes of very fine membrane known as fascia, which continuously rub against each other as various parts of the the body move. All fascia require a layer of water in between them in order to provide lubrication as various organs and tissues rub against each other. When the body is dehydrated, this lubricating layer of inter-fascial fluid dries up, producing inter-fascial friction that causes tissue inflammation and chronic body pain. This is one of the main causes of the chronic pain syndrome which so many people complain of these days, and for which they take billions of dollars worth of toxic chemical drugs to suppress, and yet most of this pain can usually be relieved simply by drinking sufficient quantities of pure alkaline water each day. If you drink specially energized waters, such as ionized micro-clustered water or oxygen water, then the therapeutic benefits of hydration become even greater and take effect faster. Proper daily hydration with good quality water is therefore the first remedy one should try for all types of chronic pain, including headaches, as well as for daytime fatigue.

The water used by most people throughout the world today carries more toxic elements into their bodies than it washes out. Typical tap water contains chlorine, fluoride, aluminium and a variety of toxic heavy metals such as lead, cadmium and nickel. This is 'dead' water, killed by chemical additives and acid elements, not the 'living' water the body requires to function properly. Most commercial bottled waters are not much better, and the minerals in the so-called 'mineral water' that's sold these days as an expensive gourmet health beverage are not in the ionized, micro-clustered form required by the cells for assimilation and utilization.

What's required here is alkaline, ionized water that has been 'restructured' into micro-cluster form. Only alkaline water can effectively neutralize acids in the blood and tissues and carry them away for excretion, and only alkaline minerals are beneficial to the body. Water that is charged with negative ions functions as a potent antioxidant to scavenge free radicals and prevent degenerative damage to the cells and tissues; negative ions also neutralize all toxic substances in the bloodstream, because all toxins in the body take on a positive charge. Water that's been restructured into micro-cluster form passes easily through cell walls and tissue membranes, quickly hydrating the whole body and delivering essential nutrients into the cells, while also flushing out and carrying away toxic wastes. Water thus plays four fundamental roles in the body: hydration, alkalization, mineralization and detoxification.

Microwater

A device has recently been developed in Japan that produces alkaline, ionized, micro-clustered water, known in health circles as microwater or 'restructured water'. It's a small machine about the size of a large dictionary that sits on the kitchen counter and attaches to any tap. First the water runs through a very fine activated charcoal filter to remove solid particles and microbes, then it enters a chamber with two titanium plates that are coated with platinum. By the process of electrolysis, all alkaline minerals held in solution in the water are drawn towards one plate, while all the acid elements, such as chlorine, fluoride and heavy metals, are drawn to the other plate. The acid water drains out an exit tube into the sink for disposal, and the alkaline water is dispensed through a spout for consumption.

In Japan, microwater has been successfully used to treat cancer, arthritis, immune dysfunction and many other debilitating conditions, and it is now beginning to catch on in the West. Dr Theodore Baroody, author of the aptly titled book *Alkalize or Die*, uses micro-clustered water as a therapeutic tool in his clinical practice, and says, 'It is my opinion that this technology will change the way in which all health care providers and the public approach their health in the coming years.' Microwater has become so popular in Japan that bars and nightclubs now make all their ice and mix all their drinks with alkaline ionized microwater, and Japanese drinkers claim that when they mix their whisky with microwater and use microwater ice cubes, they never get hangovers the next morning, regardless how much they drink at night. That's because the negatively charged alkaline microwater neutralizes the acid by-products of alcohol metabolism and flushes them out of the body before they get lodged in the liver, brain and other tissues.

The microwater technology does three things to water:

Alkalize By eliminating every molecule of acid while retaining all alkaline minerals, it alkalizes the water with beneficial minerals. These alkaline elements serve two functions: they neutralize acids and thereby restore proper pH balance to the blood and tissues; and they mineralize the cells with beneficial alkaline minerals in ionized micro-cluster form.

Ionize Elecrolysis ionizes the water molecules as well as the minerals with an extra electron, giving them a negative charge and turning them into potent antioxidants that scavenge free radicals throughout the body. Free radicals are highly reactive toxic particles produced in the body as by-products of metabolism, as well as by chemical contamination from pollutants in food, water and air. These aggressive molecular fragments chip particles from cell walls and react with bodily fluids, producing more free radicals in an escalating chain reaction that causes structural damage to internal organs, joints, skin and other bodily tissues. Negative ions immobilise free radicals by attaching to them and neutralizing their positive charge, allowing them to be flushed out of the body. Negative ions also charge each water molecule with strong anti-toxin properties that enable it to neutralize and carry away positively charged toxic molecules in the blood and tissues.

Micro-cluster This technology also breaks the alkaline minerals and the water itself into smaller micro-clusters, so that they pass more easily and swiftly into the cells and tissues to hydrate, alkalize, mineralize and detoxify the body. Ordinary water clumps in clusters of about 12 molecules each, while microwater is restructured into clusters of only 5–6 molecules. Similarly, the alkaline ionized minerals are reduced into smaller molecular clusters, so that they too pass easily into the cells to re-mineralize them.

There are many good reasons to get one of these units and use it for all of your water requirements both at home and at work, including cooking, making coffee and tea, and preparing ice cubes. During a detox programme, drinking microwater is a great way to neutralize and flush out all the toxins and acids that drain from the tissues and bodily fluids, and to quickly rehydrate the body and keep the blood alkaline. If you use microwater for all your drinking and cooking requirements at home, it provides you with an ongoing mini-detox each and every day.

Microwater is a highly efficient antioxidant, and if you drink it throughout the day, it provides continuous antioxidant activity in the blood and tissues. Since free radical damage is now commonly acknowledged in medical science as the primary cause of premature aging and tissue deterioration, drinking microwater daily can help you slow down the aging process and prevent a lot of unnecessary debilitating damage to your tissues. Many people complain that they find it difficult to drink large amounts of water, but drinking two large glasses of alkaline microwater is both easy and pleasant, because the microclusters allow it to assimilate so quickly through your stomach and into your blood and tissues. By contrast, drinking just one glass of ordinary 'dead' tap water or commercially bottled water makes your stomach feel bloated and heavy, because it just sits and pools there, like a stagnant pond, and that's why so few people like to drink water these days. Microwater solves the problem of 'hydrophobia', as well as the problem of dehydration, by making it pleasant to drink sufficient amounts of water throughout the day, and its positive effects can be felt immediately. Its alkalinity counteracts the excess stomach acidity caused by modern eating habits; its micro-clustered minerals and trace elements provide essential nutrients that are chronically deficient in modern diets; and its negative ion charge continuously scavenges free radicals and sweeps toxic substances from the bloodstream, enhancing overall vitality. All these benefits come at a cost that amounts to only a small fraction of what you'd pay for expensive nutritional and antioxidant supplements sold in health shops, and in the long run it's also much cheaper than buying bottled drinking water.

Other new technologies which enhance the blood purifying and tissue detoxifying powers of water include the Vortex Energizer and the Grander Living Water System, both of which utilize water's unique capacity to transmit energy and information into the human system, by imprinting it with healing energy frequencies and wave patterns. The Vortex Energizer, developed by the Centre for Implosion Research in England, is a small device that energizes water and counteracts the damaging influence of artificial electromagnetic fields in the environment. Drinking this activated water strengthens the human immune system, purifies the blood and protects the body from toxic contamination.

The Grander Living Water System, invented by Austrian naturalist Johann Grander, revitalizes ordinary tap water by running it through a chamber in which it is exposed to sealed cylinders of highly energized water drawn from a 5,000-year-old artesian spring in Austria. This water, which carries the natural electromagnetic properties of the earth itself, is further encoded with healing energy information by subjecting it to implosion technology and properly balanced bio-magnetic fields. As it passes through the chamber, the flowing water picks up the precise energy frequencies and polarity patterns encoded in the programmed water in the cylinders, thereby becoming identically 'informed' to perform cleansing and healing functions in the body. In addition to purifying the bloodstream and detoxifying the tissues, Grander Water imparts its bio-active energies to all the vital fluids in the body, thereby enhancing immune response, improving digestion, facilitating excretion and increasing the overall vitality and resistance of the whole system.

Seawater and sea salt

Seawater has precisely the same pH as healthy blood and contains all of the essential minerals and trace elements, in exactly the correct proportions, required by the human body. The sea is therefore an excellent source of mineral nutrients for human health, especially those rare trace elements that are generally missing in modern diets. It's also a rich source of alkalizing elements that counteract acidosis in the blood and tissues.

If you live near the ocean, one way to use seawater as a supplement is to keep a bottle of it in your refrigerator and drink a few millilitres each day, diluted in a glass of pure water. Dr Norman Walker, who lived to the age of 116 by periodically detoxifying his body, keeping his blood and tissues at proper pH balance and eating properly, drank small amounts of seawater daily in order to ensure that his bloodstream contained all of the essential elements, known and not yet known, required by the blood and cells. If you're doing a detox programme at a health resort near the ocean, this is a good way to help neutralize all the acid wastes that are released from your tissues by detox, and to provide your body with all the essential minerals it needs to support the detox process. It's important, however, to make sure that the water is drawn from clear, unpolluted parts of the ocean, not from contaminated coastal waters. One way to do this – if you are near the sea – is to ask someone on a fishing or diving boat to haul 4 litres of clean seawater from deeper offshore waters.

Another way to tap into the sea as a source of alkalizing minerals and essential trace elements is to use whole, unrefined sea salt for all of your culinary requirements and also as a nutritional supplement. The best choice here is what's known as Celtic sea salt. 'Celtic' refers to an ancient northern European method of harvesting whole sea salt that it still practised along the Brittany coast in northern France today. This method retains all of the essential elements in the salt, as well as the important trace elements contained in the brine. The brine, also known as bittern or 'mother liquor', is the thick residual fluid that remains in the salt pans after wind and sun have evaporated the water and the salt has been collected. Much of this brine remains in the harvested sea salt, giving it the characteristic light grey colour and slight dampness that distinguishes genuine Celtic sea salt from ordinary refined forms of sea salt. The word Celtic designates this sort of whole, unrefined, naturally harvested sea salt, which is very different from the so-called sea salt commonly found in most supermarkets today. Commercially refined sea salt is heated and bleached, and often treated with additives, in order to make it snow-white and to prevent clumping, but this process also strips the salt of many of its essential nutritional elements, especially the vital trace elements contained in the bittern.

Celtic sea salt contains 84 minerals and trace elements, including every one that is essential to human health. Its light grey colour and moist crystals are the identifying traits which indicate the presence of the bittern in the salt. Besides providing all of the essential minerals required by the body, it bestows some specific benefits that are particularly helpful for detoxification and rejuvenation. It contains organic iodine, which, unlike the refined iodine added to industrially processed table salt, protects the body from harmful radiation in the environment and radioactive fallout in the atmosphere. The micro-minerals in Celtic sea salt provide the adrenal and pituitary glands with precisely the elements they require to sustain balanced secretions of vital hormones. Studies have shown that when refined table salt is used, secretions of the adrenal and pituitary glands are measurably reduced, resulting in low vitality, low motivation and low libido.

The denatured, industrially refined table salt that most people in the world use today does more harm to the body than it does good. This salt has been robbed of its synergistic minerals, trace elements and other co-factors, leaving a denatured white substance that is 99.9 per cent sodium choloride. Doctors today often advise people to drastically reduce their salt intake in order to prevent high blood pressure, but this advice applies only to the deleterious effects of industrially processed table salt, which contains an unnaturally high ratio of sodium and no synergistic co-factors to counter-balance the excess sodium. Furthermore, the sodium in refined table salt is hardened, and it therefore remains lodged in the body for an excessively long time, which is why it causes blood pressure problems. The sodium in Celtic sea salt retains its natural pliant form, is less concentrated and drains out of the body quickly. Furthermore, some of the trace elements contained in the bittern automatically neutralize and flush out excess sodium from the blood and tissues, thereby preventing it from causing any problems.

One way to use Celtic sea salt as an alkalizing mineral supplement is simply to dissolve about ⅓ teaspoon in a glass of water and drink it. This is also very helpful when you experience excess acidity in the stomach. Another way is to reconstitute the bittern or 'mother liquor' from whole Celtic sea salt, which is richly permeated with bittern, and use this as a supplement. To make your own bittern, place 2.25–4.5 kg of coarse light grey Celtic sea salt in a clean, unbleached cotton bag and tie the bag shut with a piece of string. Fill a large pot with pure spring water, and soak the bag of salt in the water for 3–5 minutes. Then hang the soaked bag of salt over a ceramic or glass bowl (but not metal), and let all of the fluid drip into the bowl. Funnel it into clean glass bottles, and take about 30 ml of this reconstituted bittern, diluted in pure water, once or twice a day.

Magnesium is one of the macro-minerals that is most required for human health, but today more than half the population of the world suffers a critical deficiency of magnesium, including people in the richest, most highly developed countries, such as America and Western Europe. Magnesium deficiency is a major contributing factor to heart disease, and studies in America have shown that more than half of the fatal heart attacks there could probably have been be avoided if adequate magnesium supplementation had been administered in time. A shortage of magnesium contributes to depression, insomnia, irritability and other problems related to central nervous system dysfunction. Magnesium is also one of the most important nutrients required by the body during the detox process, because magnesium is an essential element for the production of a multitude of alkaline enzymes that are required for the detoxification process. It is therefore a good idea to include some form of magnesium supplementation in any detox programme, as well as in daily life.

You can prepare an excellent magnesium supplement your-self at home, using Celtic sea salt and magnesium chloride hexahydrate. Dissolve 8 g of Celtic sea salt in 1 litre of cold water, and seal tightly in a bottle with a cap. Then dissolve 12 g of magnesium chloride hexahydrate in 1 litre of cold water, and cap it in a clean bottle as well. To use, mix one part of the salt solution with five parts of the magnesium solution and three or four parts of your favourite fruit or vegetable juice, or herbal tea, to make one full cup (250 ml). Drink one cup in the morning and another in the evening for a period of 10–15 days, in order to correct conditions related to magnesium deficiency, and as a support for any detox programme. For ordinary use as a daily dietary supplement, one glass in the morning is sufficient.

While we are on the topic of internal salt water therapy, let's take a quick look at an ancient Indian technique for detoxifying and restoring the delicate tissues of the sinus cavity. Known as the Neti nasal douche, this method employs whole sea salt dissolved in warm water to gently wash the sinuses and flush out dust, smoke, air pollutants and other toxic residues that become lodged in the sinus cavities. It's a highly refreshing cleanse that greatly improves nasal breathing, fully restores the sense of smell and detoxifies the convoluted passages of the sinuses.

To do the Neti nasal douche, put about ⅔ teaspoon of Celtic sea salt into a small ceramic tea pot of about 350 ml capacity. Add warm water at about body temperature and stir to completely dissolve the salt. Bend forwards, or kneel down, place the spout of the tea pot firmly into the left nostril, then tilt the head slowly to the right, until the water starts flowing into the left nostril, through the left sinus passage, and back out through the right sinus passage and right nostril, in a steady stream. When about half the solution is used, switch over to the other side and do the same thing. When you've finished the solution, bend forwards and rock your head up and down, then from side to side, while snorting air out your nostrils to blow residual water from the nasal passages.

Oxygen water

Less than 200 years ago, the earth's atmosphere contained about 38 per cent oxygen. Today, oxygen constitutes only about 19 per cent of the air we breathe, half of its former level, and a lot less than that in polluted inner cities. Oxygen deficiency has therefore become a common condition throughout the world, and it's a major contributing factor in toxaemia, immune deficiency, cancer and most chronic degeneration conditions. Since the air we breathe delivers only half the oxygen we require per breath, it's very helpful to provide an additional form of oxygen supplementation during detox, and one of the most effective ways is to use oxygenated water.

Besides its essential role as a fuel for metabolism, oxygen is also the great cleansing agent of the body. All toxins must first combine with oxygen in order to be carried out of the cells and tissues for excretion. Oxygen kills bacteria and viruses, neutralizes toxins, and purifies the blood, tissues and individual cells. Unlike antibiotics, however, which kill friendly as well as harmful bacteria, oxygen kills only the harmful anaerobic bacteria that invade the inside of the body, without damaging the beneficial bacteria in the bowels and other tissues. Brian Goulet, a health practitioner who utilizes oxygen therapy in his clinical practice, says, 'Rubble, garbage, toxins, refuse, debris, and anything useless, are destroyed by oxygen and carried out of the system. Just as a clean house holds little interest to passing flies, likewise any oxygen-rich body is a difficult fortress to assail.' Molecular biologist Dr Stephen Levine believes that oxygen deficiency could be the beginning phase of immune deficiency syndrome. Says he, 'We can look at oxygen deficiency as the single great cause of all diseases. It is believed and supported by a great deal of research, that a shortage of oxygen in the blood could very well be the starting point for the breakdown of the immune system.'

One of the swiftest ways to oxygenate water to produce an oxygen supplement is to put a few drops of hydrogen peroxide into a glass of pure water. Hydrogen peroxide has the same molecular structure as water, except that it has an extra oxygen molecule. When dissolved in water, each molecule of hydrogen peroxide breaks down to produce one molecule of ordinary water and one molecule of free oxygen. These extra molecules of free oxygen enter the bloodstream and circulate throughout the tissues, thereby enriching the entire body with additional supplies of detoxifying oxygen. When you first start using hydrogen peroxide as an oxygen supplement, it's advisable to consult a health professional for some specific guidance.

During detox, a small daily dose of hydrogen peroxide provides the blood with an extra boost of oxygen to deal with the overload of toxins that are released into the bloodstream from the tissues. In addition, you may take daily doses of this oxygenated water to protect yourself from the flu and other contagious diseases during epidemics. In the autumn of 1983, in the midst of an avian flu outbreak that killed over 11 million chickens in America, about one million chickens were given small amounts of hydrogen peroxide in their drinking water, and not a single one of these birds died of the disease.

Another effective way to oxygenate water is to bubble ozone gas through it, but to do that, you must have a special ozone machine. Some spas and health resorts now have these devices. Drinking water treated with ozone releases even more free oxygen into the bloodstream than water treated with hydrogen peroxide, and this makes it a very useful item for internal cleansing purposes. As Dr George Freibott of the International Association for Oxygen Therapy states, 'Oxygen is a powerful detoxifier, and when its quantity is deficient, toxins begin to devastate body functions and deplete the body of life-giving energy.'

One of the most remarkable oxygen supplements on the market today is a specially formulated solution of 'heavy water' (deuterium sulphate) known as ESF, which stands for Everett Storey Formula, named after the American nuclear scientist who invented it during the 1950s. This product is sold throughout the world under licence from the company that holds the patent, using various different brand-names, including Cellfood, Liquid Life ESF, Hydrocell, Cellogen and Hydroxygen.

ESF is based on a patented 'split water' technology. What it does is split a very small amount of the water molecules in your body to release one molecule of free oxygen and two molecules of free hydrogen, which enter the blood and permeate the cells. As we have already noted, oxygen is one of nature's most potent detoxifiers, and oxygen levels in the air we breathe, which is our primary source, have dropped by half over the past 200 years. ESF therefore serves to correct this oxygen deficiency by providing the body with a constant internal stream of free oxygen released from water. It also releases free hydrogen, which is an essential element for producing energy, repairing cells and maintaining strong immune response. ESF contains microscopic, ionized forms of 78 vital minerals, 34 essential enzymes and 17 important amino acids, which are all carried into the cells along with the oxygen and hydrogen. ESF is therefore both a potent nutritional supplement and a highly effective detoxifying agent.

ESF should be taken three times daily (early morning, afternoon and night) in order to ensure a steady stream of free oxygen and hydrogen in the blood and tissues. For detox programmes, or to help cure specific diseases, eight drops of ESF taken three times daily in a glass of plain water or juice is an effective dosage. For ordinary use as a daily supplement, five drops three times a day is sufficient. To order this product, please refer to the section on 'Suppliers' in Appendix 2.

External uses: hydrotherapy

During detox, the skin must bear an extra heavy burden as an excretory outlet for toxic wastes, and it can easily get damaged and become blemished from contact with all the toxins that pass through the pores. The skin therefore needs special attention while the body is detoxifying itself in order to prevent toxic damage and to facilitate the rapid elimination of all toxins that are driven from the lymph, blood and tissues out to the surface of the skin.

It should be noted that, unlike the interior of the body, which should be slightly alkaline, the exterior surface of the skin should have a slightly acid mantle to protect the body from invasion by external pathogens. While the microbes which invade the interior of the body are anaerobic and thrive in acid environments, those which attack the exterior surface are aerobic and cannot tolerate an acid environment, which is why the skin is meant to have a slightly acidic pH value. Most people wash away this acid mantle on a daily basis, by using commercial bath soaps and shampoos, all of which contain strong alkaline detergents. This renders the skin vulnerable to infections, rashes and other irritations. It's therefore advisable to cut down on the use of commercial bath soaps and shampoos, or else to switch to milder varieties made only from pure vegetable, nut and essential oils, without chemical additives. Another solution is to keep a bucket of the ionized acid water discharged from a microwater ionizing unit in the bathroom, and rinse your skin and hair with a few cups of this water after finishing your shower or bath. Since this acid water has been filtered, ionized and reduced to micro-clusters, the same as the alkaline portion that you consume internally, it too is an extremely pure and potent therapeutic water, but serves instead as an antiseptic acidifying agent for external use on the skin and hair.

The best way to protect your skin from damage and accelerate the excretion of toxic wastes through the pores during detox is to soak your body, or even just your feet, in hot water laced with sea salt or Epsom salts and a few drops of detoxifying essential oils. If you don't have time for a full body soak, or if you don't have a bathtub at home, just soaking your feet and ankles in a basin of hot salt water is also very effective, for it draws toxic wastes through the lymph channels down to the feet and facilitates their excretion out of the body into the water.

Hot salt water baths

The most popular way to prepare a hot salt water bath today is to add a cup or two of Epsom salts to a bathtub full of hot water. Epsom salts are various forms of magnesium salts, and these are particularly effective for detoxifcation purposes because they stimulate lymph drainage and draw toxins out through the pores by osmosis.

You can also use coarse grey Celtic sea salt to prepare a hot salt water bath for detox purposes, as it contains dozens of beneficial micro-minerals and trace elements in the bittern. Just add 1.35 kg of grey Celtic sea salt plus 450 g of magnesium chloride hexahydrate to a bathtub full of hot water, and soak in it for about half an hour. The higher the salinity of the bath water, the stronger the power of osmosis that draws the toxins out through the skin, so for intensive detox purposes you need to use a greater quantity of sea salt, and add magnesium chloride for an extra boost of lymphatic detox. For ordinary salt water bathing, 450–900 g of grey Celtic sea salt on its own is sufficient to cleanse the skin and mildly detoxify the system – the magnesium chloride can be omitted.

A particularly potent form of sea salt comes from the Dead Sea in the Jordan Valley. At 400 metres below sea level, the Dead Sea is the lowest spot on the surface of the earth, and it produces a bath salt that is extremely rich in medicinal minerals and natural detoxifying agents. This bath salt, which is available from health product suppliers, has both detoxifying as well as healing properties, and hot Dead Sea salt baths provide highly beneficial support for the skin during detox.

Another useful skin detox product from the Dead Sea is therapeutic mineral mud. Dead Sea mud has amazing cleansing and healing powers, and it seems to work on both the physical biochemical level as well as the energetic electromagnetic level. To use Dead Sea mud for detox, put a sufficient amount of mud into a bowl and place the bowl in hot water to heat the mud. Smear the mud thickly over the affected part of the skin, cover with cling film or cellophane, and secure with medical tape. Leave it there for about an hour, then wash off the mud, and take a hot Dead Sea salt bath. One woman in Australia reports that she cured herself of breast cancer and completely eliminated the tumours by applying Dead Sea mud packs and soaking in Dead Sea salt baths repeatedly over a period of several months. While such evidence is often discounted as 'anecdotal', it's nevertheless a documented fact that it happened, and if such a cure can work once, it can certainly work again.

The therapeutic benefits of hot salt water baths may be further enhanced by the addition of essential oils that have detoxifying and healing properties. Since these oils are also highly aromatic, some of their therapeutic essence is absorbed through the sinuses and lungs as the volatile vapours rise from the hot bath water. The oil of grapefruit seed and peel is a particularly good choice for helping to detoxify the lymphatic system. Sage and rosemary both have potent tissue cleansing properties, and peppermint oil may also be used for detox purposes. If you're feeling enervated and 'uptight', try adding a few drops of frankincense oil to your hot salt water bath, or a dash of lavender. Keep a variety of these essential oils in the bathroom, and experiment with different combinations for various conditions.

Another way to enhance the therapeutic power of bathwater

is to use a jacuzzi or whirlpool tub. The water jets create a soothing, healing energy pulse deep within the body as a result of the 'piezoelectric effect' of the vibrations in the water on the crystaline structures in bones, glands, connective tissue and bodily fluids. The vibratory stimulation also activates lymph drainage and boosts micro-circulation in the tissues just below the skin, thereby facilitating elimination of toxic wastes through the pores.

Bathing in the sea

If you live near the ocean, or stay at a health resort by the sea, daily plunges are another good way to provide your body with saline detox hydrotherapy. Seawater contains all of the medicinal minerals and cleansing elements found in sea salt, and sea bathing therefore allows the skin to detoxify and repair itself, albeit not as intensively as in a hot bath containing high concentrations of mineral salts. Again, be sure that the sea is clean before you jump in, otherwise you'll come out even more toxic than before. Avoid harbour waters and areas where raw sewage is discharged.

Another benefit of bathing daily in open seawater is that the ocean, which has its own vast electromagnetic energy field, naturally recharges and rebalances the human energy system whenever the body is submerged in it. This contributes significantly to the detoxification and regeneration process, and accelerates healing. In addition, the air along ocean shores is highly charged with negative ions, which also help detoxify the blood and tissues and facilitate rapid elimination of wastes. Finally, the rhythmic force of waves and currents in the ocean provides a gentle massage to the entire body, providing similar therapeutic effects as those discussed for whirlpool baths. Added together, these various benefits transform a daily dip in the ocean into an effective and pleasant therapeutic activity.

No doubt that's one reason so many spas and health resorts are located by the sea.

Mineral hot springs

Since time immemorial, throughout Asia as well as the Western world, soaking in steamy mineral water baths at natural hot spring sources has been a traditional way of relaxing, cleansing and healing the body. Today, this ancient custom is still widely practised as a health regimen in East Asia, particularly in Japan, Korea and Taiwan, whose mountain ranges are riddled with natural hot springs. In Japan, the mountainous southern island of Kyushu is the place to go for traditional hot spring spas, many of which feature charming old Japanese inns with all the traditional amenities. In Korea, there are numerous hot spring resorts in the mountains along the southern and eastern coastline, and in Taiwan, the entire island steams with over a hundred hot spring sources, from the well developed traditional hot spring resorts of Peitou in the north to the rustic alfresco spas in the central highlands and southeast coastal region. Some of these hot springs have been operated as health spas and rest retreats for hundreds of years.

Since hot springs are usually located in rugged mountain settings that often feature waterfalls as well, a few words on the purifying power of falling water are in order here. Waterfalls produce a powerful, pulsing energy field that radiates for many metres, and the effect of this vibrant field on the human energy system, when one sits tranquilly at rest by a waterfall, is to detoxify and rebalance the entire system. Simply sitting quietly beside a big waterfall, and cultivating a calm state of mental serenity and physical relaxation, quickly clears blockages and corrects imbalances in the human energy field, and this in turn activates cleansing and healing responses in the nervous and endocrine systems. In addition, the air around waterfalls is richly charged with negative ions. Breathing this air saturates the blood with negative ion energy, which acts as a powerful anti-oxidant to scavenge free radicals and neutralize toxins in the bloodstream, tissues and cells This detox effect is swift, and it reaches the deepest tissues of the body. This form of hydrotherapy works on both the physical and energetic levels and may be utilized as an effective support for any detox programme. Indeed, 'sitting still doing nothing' beside a waterfall is an ancient Taoist way of practising meditation, so you may combine your meditation practice with your hydrotherapy and reap a richer harvest from both.

Herbal steam power

Among the most effective and pleasant ways of all to detox is to use traditional Thai herbal steam therapy, which is one of the most efficient methods of ridding the body of toxic wastes through the skin and lungs. It's basically the same set-up as any ordinary steamroom system, except that highly aromatic medicinal herbs are added to the water in the boiler to produce a therapeutic herbal steam that engages both skin and lungs in the detox process. This is also a form of aromatherapy, but instead of just sniffing the aromatic essence released in the air through your nose, you immerse your entire body in it and breathe in hot damp vapour that carries the medicinal aromatic essences of the herbs deeply into your lungs, where they quickly absorb into the bloodstream and circulate directly to every tissue of the body, delivering their therapeutic powers to each and every cell. At the same time, the hot steam opens the pores and allows the herbal vapours to enter the skin to draw toxins out with the sweat. Thai herbal steam simultaneously cleanses the body from the inside and the outside, providing a doubly detoxifying effect as well as a very relaxing, soothing experience.

At the beginning of the 20th century, there were hundreds of herbal steam facilities all over Thailand. Every town and village had them, and many were located on the premises of Buddhist temples, where traditional Thai medicine is still taught and practised by monks today. Herbal steam served as a primary form of healing and health care, with specific formulas for every disease and condition. Today, these herbal remedies have been replaced by Western pharmaceutical drugs, and public health in Thailand has diminished proportionately as a result. Nevertheless, you can still find traditional herbal steam facilities in most of Thailand's cities and resort areas, and you can also set up your own steam room at home.

More than 70 different aromatic herbs are used in traditional Thai steam therapy, but the primary ones are lemongrass, kaffir lime, ginger root, galanga root, basil, cinnamon, rosemary, thyme, pepper and mint. In addition, you may also use aromatic medicinal herbs from other regions of the world, particularly those known for their cleansing, relaxing and rejuvenating properties such as lavender, lemon balm and sage. The exact proportions are not particularly important, and they may be blended according to personal preference. As to quantity, that depends upon how strong you wish to make the steam and how big the boiler is in your steamer system. Generally speaking, you might use a total of 200–250 g of mixed fresh herbs, or 100–125 g of mixed dried herbs, for a medium sized steam boiler of 20–40 litres capacity. Fresh and dried herbs may also be mixed together in the same batch. The lemongrass should preferably be fresh rather than dried in order to derive maximum benefit from this refreshing, relaxing, highly aromatic herb. Fill the steam boiler with water and let it come to a full boil before adding the herbs, which should be coarsely chopped. The herbs may be added directly to the boiling water, or else placed inside a cloth spice bag and tied shut with a string, before being dropped into the boiling water. You may experiment with a variety of different blends until you discover the ones that suit you best. Meanwhile, as a general guideline, several classic combinations that are still commonly used in traditional Thai herbal steam therapy today are given on page 324 in the Recipes and Formulas section in Appendix 1.

To use an herbal steam bath for detox therapy, first drink a few cups of hot herbal tea that has cleansing or relaxing properties, such as camomile, peppermint, sage or ginger. Then enter the steamroom and sit quietly inside for about 20 minutes, breathing deeply through the nose. Next, leave the steamroom and take a plunge in a cool pool, or stand under a cold shower, to cool off the body, rinse sweat from the skin, close the pores and stimulate the lymph and endocrine systems. Relax for 5–10 minutes, then repeat the process two or three more times. When you're finished, be sure to drink at least two large glasses of alkaline water to rehydrate your tissues and remineralize your cellular fluids.

Water shortage

Today, the supply of pure, naturally balanced water is shrinking at an alarming rate. The water situation has got so bad that many people now depend on bottled water for their daily drinking supplies, because the water provided by most municipal water utilities is so overloaded with chemicals that it makes your body even more toxic.

Water's incredible solvent properties are a two-edged sword. On the one hand, water is required to dissolve and transport essential nutrients, trace elements and herbal essences into the cells and tissues; water vapour can carry healing herbal energies into the lungs and skin; and water can neutralize and flush away virtually any toxin in the body. On the other hand, this also means that water dissolves any toxic substance to which it is exposed in the environment, holds it in solution, and transports it wherever it goes. Thus, the more toxic the environment becomes, the more poisonous the world's water supply gets. Regardless of whether you use it internally or externally, water can either harm you by bringing dissolved toxins in solution into your body, or else heal you by dissolving toxins that are already imbedded in your system and carrying them out of the body as liquid waste. It all depends on the original quality of the water you use, how well you purify it, and whether you 'programme' it to nourish, cleanse and heal your body.

Most of the water on the earth today has been seriously polluted and acidified by various artificial means, such as industrial waste, sewage and chemicals such as chlorine and fluoride. The only way to purify and alkalize it for consumption is to use special technology that makes it fit for human health and healing. When used for intensive detox purposes, water may be specifically programmed in the various ways discussed in this chapter in order to enhance its hydrating and alkalizing properties, increase its cleansing and detoxifying effects, and amplify its antioxidant activity.

It's also important to remember that when taking water internally for detox purposes as well as for ordinary daily consumption, quantity is every bit as important as quality. Water can only work to cleanse and heal your body if you drink sufficient quantities each day to keep your blood and tissues consistently well hydrated and to fully replenish the water lost with the excretion of wastes. In order to prevent dehydration and keep your bodily fluids fresh, you need to drink about two litres (6–8 glasses) of pure water per day.

CHAPTER 3

Physiotherapy: Massage and Soft Exercise

Stagnation of bodily fluids due to insufficient movement is one of the great afflictions of modern life and a major contributing factor to chronic toxaemia. The more 'convenient' life becomes – with cars to replace feet, machines to wash clothes, lifts to avoid stairs and motors to perform virtually every other chore – the more sedentary people will become and the less they will exercise their bodies. Like stagnant ponds, their bodily fluids will become inert and turbid, losing vitality and the capacity to support life. In the section on health in the Confucian classic *Spring and Autumn Annals*, compiled over 2,000 years ago, it is written, 'if the body does not move, essence [vital fluids] does not flow. When essence does not flow, energy stagnates.' And when energy stagnates, the whole system loses power, and the first function to fail is the body's ability to cleanse and repair itself.

The human body was designed by nature to move, not to remain perpetually inert and immobile, and bodily fluids were meant to flow, not to sit and stagnate. Some of these vital fluids, such as lymph, depend entirely on body movements for their own mobility. When you're watching television or sitting at a desk, riding in a car or standing in a lift, your lymph stands still and your blood slows down, and whenever this happens, waste drainage halts and toxins accumulate rapidly in the blood and tissues. Insufficient exercise also stiffens the joints and tightens the tendons, congests the bowels and reduces metabolic efficiency. Activity is the principal attribute of energy and of life itself, while inertia and stagnation pave the way for decay and death.

During detox, it's especially important to keep your blood, lymph and other bodily fluids flowing freely, to keep your joints loose and limber, to stretch your tendons and other connective tissue, and to stimulate your organs and glands. There is a tendency during detox to remain inert and inactive, because the detox process makes your body feel tired, weak and sluggish as the toxins are released continuously into the bloodstream for elimination. However, if you don't move your body and keep your fluids flowing, the released toxins remain circulating in your bloodstream for a much longer period of time, making you feel even worse and prolonging both the discomfort and the length of the detox process.

Fortunately, if you're too lazy or too tired to mobilize your own body and move your own blood and lymph during detox, you can pay someone else to do it for you with therapeutic massage, which kneads toxins from the tissues, activates lymph drainage, stimulates glandular secretions, calms the nervous system and tones the joints, muscles and tendons. If you cannot afford professional massage every day, or if it's not available, you may apply self-massage techniques instead to facilitate the detox process and prevent stagnation. Alternatively, you could practise some form of traditional Asian 'soft' style exercise, such as yoga, Tai Chi or *chi gung*, or simply go for a stroll or a swim every day, to keep your body loose and limber, to stretch and tone your tissues, and to keep the 'cleansing waters' of your bodily fluids flowing freely.

Massage

The Chinese term for massage translates literally into English as 'press and rub', reflecting its two main techniques: deep tissue pressure, followed by shallow surface rubbing, applied alternately. The deep pressure stimulates vital points along the meridiens and dislodges toxic deposits in the tissues; the rubbing then scatters the released toxins and facilitates their drainage through the blood and lymph. There are a variety of different styles of traditional Asian massage, and most of them work with a combination of deep tissue pressure and soothing surface palpation.

You may enhance the therapeutic benefits of detox massage by thoroughly washing your body (or having a herbal steam) before the massage, in order to remove dirt, oil, sweat and toxic residues from your skin. Eliminating this greasy layer of dust, dead cells and dried perspiration from the surface of your skin facilitates the interaction and exchange of energy between your body and the massage therapist's hands, and this in turn amplifies the therapeutic benefits of the massage and corrects imbalances in your energy field. It's important to rest quietly and remain completely relaxed throughout the duration of a therapeutic massage. Don't allow yourself to be disturbed by loud music, blaring televisions, urgent phone calls or any other invasive distraction, and abstain from carrying on a conversation while you're receiving massage therapy. Energy always follows wherever you aim your attention, so if you focus attention on external sensory distractions during a massage, your energy will flow out to those distractions and dissipate externally. On the other hand, if you focus your attention internally, shining it like a spotlight on the parts of the body that are being massaged, your energy will flow there instead, magnifying the therapeutic power of the massage on that part of the body. Last but not least, don't forget to drink one or two large glasses of pure alkaline water immediately after every therapeutic massage, especially during a detox programme. This is necessary to quickly dissolve, flush out and excrete the avalanche of toxins that deep tissue massage releases into the blood and lymph from every part of the body.

Traditional Thai massage

Thai massage originated in India, but over the centuries it has also adopted some techniques from China, such as applying acupressure to vital points along the energy meridiens. It is one of the most comprehensive and effective therapeutic massage systems in the world, combining deep tissue massage, yoga stretches applied to your body by the therapist, acupressure therapy, joint and spine manipulation, and direct stimulation of the endocrine glands. Even the force of gravity is employed to mobilize the flow of vital fluids by holding the body in various upside-down postures. Another manoeuvre unique to Thai massage is the artery block, whereby the major arteries that feed blood into the legs are blocked shut by manual pressure for 30–45 seconds, then suddenly released. This brings a strong wave of blood rushing warmly down through the legs, sweeping loose plaque and other debris from the walls of these arteries and providing a big boost to circulation throughout the system.

A session of traditional Thai massage, which is known as *nuat boran* and is still widely practised in Thailand today, should last for at least an hour, preferably two or three. Some of the older, classically trained massage masters in Thailand refuse to do a session of less than two hours, because this therapy was designed to slowly and very systematically detoxify, tone and rebalance the entire human system, including all the organs, glands and tissues of the physical body, as well as the channels, chakras and fields of the energy body. This takes time, and since some of the techniques are quite powerful, such as the artery block and the spinal stretches, they cannot be applied quickly in rapid succession. Instead, strong and gentle techniques are applied alternately, gradually preparing the body for the deeper techniques and giving it time to adjust and rebalance itself after each major shift.

Again, don't forget to drink one or two large glasses of pure water after a Thai massage, as well as after any therapeutic massage. Deep tissue work releases a huge load of toxic residues stored in the body and dumps them into the bloodstream and lymph channels for elimination; if you don't drink plenty of water to wash them out afterwards, these toxins accumulate rapidly in the bloodstream and cause unpleasant side effects.

Chinese tui-na *massage*

One of the most ancient forms of therapeutic massage is Chinese *tui-na*, literally 'press and rub', which is done with the ball of the thumb, or sometimes with the knuckles of the index and middle fingers. *Tui-na* massage is performed with a single press of the thumb or knuckle, pushing deeply into the tissues, then releasing the pressure and immediately rubbing the surface with circular motion to disperse stagnant energy. This pressing and rubbing therapy is applied repeatedly along the entire length of specific energy meridiens and nerve channels associated with the organs and tissues that require treatment. Stagnant organs and toxic tissues are activated by the deep pressure along the meridiens and nerves which control them, stimulating them to discharge their toxins, recharge their cells, replenish their fluids and rebalance their functions. The deep pressure and rhythmic rubbing gradually kneads toxic residues loose from the tissues and drives them into the lymphatic system for disposal.

Since blood vessels and lymph channels follow the same basic pathways through the body as meridiens and nerves, *tui-na* therapy stimulates blood circulation and lymph drainage as well.

This facilitates swift elimination of the toxins and acid wastes discharged from the organs and other tissues.

Tui-na massage is particularly effective for dislodging impacted toxins from nerve tissue and pushing them into the lymph channels for elimination. As noted earlier, some of the most hazardous toxic substances in the body, such as heavy metals and inorganic chemicals, have a particular affinity for nerve tissue due to its electromagnetic potential. The body's natural cleansing mechanisms cannot easily eliminate these heavy toxins, and so they cling to nerve tissues, gradually becoming embedded there and causing all kinds of maladies and malfunctions of the nervous system. *Tui-na* massage applied along the entire length of the neck and spine, and down along the major nerves of the arms and legs, loosens and releases clumps of toxic deposits from the nerve tissues, allowing them to be dissolved and carried away for excretion in the blood and lymph. When the deep tissue pressure is released and followed by circular rubbing on the surface, fresh blood and energy flow into the tissues, repairing and re-charging nerves damaged by long-term toxicity.

Some *tui-na* therapists begin each session with 15–20 minutes of work applied entirely to the four branches of the bladder meridien, which run up along the spine, with two parallel channels on each side. This relaxes the internal organs, switches the nervous system into the healing mode of the parasympathetic branch, and releases tension from the muscles that support the spinal cord. These branches of the bladder meridien pass through the thick, tough bands of muscle that surround the spinal cord. In most people, these muscles are usually tight as springs with nervous tension, which compresses the upper vertebrae and inhibits the passage of nerve signals through the spinal cord and out to the organs and glands. This tension in the nerves and muscles of the spine also keeps the autonomic nervous system locked into the hyperactive 'fight or flight' responses of the sympathetic branch, thereby blocking detoxification and healing responses. By applying alternating deep tissue pressure and circular rubbing along the full length of the bladder meridiens on both sides of the spine, tension in the spinal muscles is gradually released and the entire spinal cord and all the vertebrae and surrounding connective tissues gradually relax, switching the nervous system over to the calm, healing mode of the parasympathetic branch and allowing the nerves to communicate freely with the organs and endocrine system to activate cleansing and healing responses throughout the system.

There's a special branch of *tui-na* massage in TCM called *hsiao-er tui na*, literally 'little children's *tui-na*', developed entirely for paediatric application. Most children rebel at taking bitter herbal concoctions, and they buck like broncos if a doctor tries to stick an acupuncture needle in their bodies. Paediatric *tui-na* was thus developed as a special branch of TCM to provide an effective means of applying medical therapy that children will accept. To make it even more acceptable for children, soothing aromatic oils are usually applied to the skin as well to increase the therapeutic benefits of the massage and produce a more pleasant sensation. Children are far more responsive to touch than adults, and they usually don't carry the psychic tensions that tighten the tissues of adult bodies. A relatively lighter touch may therefore be used on children's bodies than on adults, making the therapy even less invasive. Due to the softness and sensitivity of children's growing bodies therapeutic results are usually swift and effective. A weekly or monthly 'tune-up' with paediatric *tui-na* massage by a qualified therapist is an excellent preventive regimen for keeping young children's systems healthy and strong and counteracting the toxicity which junk food and environmental pollution produce in children today.

Japanese shiatsu *massage*

Shiatsu is a traditional Japanese therapy based on even older Chinese acupressure techniques, whereby the thumb or a knuckle is used to apply deep pressure to various acupuncture points, in order to produce a specific therapeutic effect in the organs associated with those points. This technique is especially effective when applied by a therapist who has developed the ability to 'emit energy' (*fa chi*) through his or her hands, thereby boosting the therapeutic benefits of the acupressure by transferring a 'turbo-charge' of healing energy directly into the patient's energy system. In recent years, both *shiatsu* and traditional Thai massage have come to the attention of alternative health care providers in Europe and North America, and many aspiring young healers from the Western world now come to Thailand and Japan in order to learn these ancient healing arts under the tutelage of accomplished masters, then return to their home countries to practise professionally. If you're doing a detox programme in an area where you can find a qualified practitioner of *shiatsu* or traditional Thai massage, you can accelerate the pace and reduce the discomfort of the detox process by having a daily treatment.

Traditional Asian foot massage

All Asian healing traditions include a special form of therapeutic massage applied exclusively to the terminals of major energy meridiens and nerve channels located in the feet. In the West, this form of foot therapy is called reflexology, but it is not nearly as well developed nor as effective as the ancient Asian method, which has been practised continuously throughout the East for thousands of years.

The techniques of traditional Asian foot massage are similar to the deep tissue pressing and surface rubbing used in *tui-na*, applied exclusively to vital points on the major meridiens and nerve channels that terminate in the feet. Six of the 12 primary organ-energy meridiens have terminals in the feet – spleen, liver, kidneys, stomach, bladder and gall bladder – and the main branches of the autonomic nervous system also have roots there. By stimulating specific points on the feet with deep tissue pressure, specific therapeutic effects may be produced in the related organs and glands of the body.

In TCM, cramped and misshapen feet are seen as a primary cause of chronic dysfunction in the internal organs and glands connected to the nerve and energy channels in the feet. These terminals are literally crushed by hardened tissues and bone deformities in the feet. The liver and kidneys, for example, which are responsible for filtering toxins from the blood, cannot properly perform their cleansing functions when the energy meridiens and nerve endings which regulate them are pinched and blocked in the feet. Consequently, toxic wastes accumulate in the blood and tissues, and bodily fluids become increasingly acidic, producing a state of chronic toxaemia that sets the stage for the onset of disease and degeneration. Deep acupressure applied to blocked nerves and meridiens on the soles of the feet triggers a massive internal cleansing response in the related organs, particularly the liver and kidneys. Particularly toxic individuals will sometimes run to the nearest toilet to pass up to a litre of coffee-coloured urine immediately after their first treatment, or to purge their bowels with a bout of diarrhoea, and a foul odour often exudes from the skin as toxins are driven out through the pores. Clearly, this is a powerful detox therapy.

Dr Lee Shih-min, a doctor from Taiwan trained in modern Western medicine, has in recent years drawn a lot of serious professional attention to this ancient Chinese healing art in America. At the University of Southern California's medical center, where he practised Western medicine for many years, he was frequently exposed to the invasive and often counterproductive methods of modern allopathic medicine and radical surgery. After a while, he says, he 'got so tired of all the needles, knives and drugs' that he started studying the ancient ways of traditional Chinese medicine in search of better methods. There he discovered foot therapy and started practising it as a side-line in his own clinic. Before long, he gained a reputation for producing 'medical miracles', and foot therapy soon became his main line, as more and more doctors and surgeons at the medical centre referred their 'hopeless cases' to him as a last resort. More often than not, he completely cured them. Initially sceptical, his medical colleagues themselves now go to him for treatment, and it can take months to get an appointment. Fortunately, Dr Lee is training a new generation of therapists in this powerful detoxification and healing technique, and hopefully it will soon become more widely available.

If you're travelling in Thailand these days, you'll notice dozens of new foot massage salons in every major city and resort area. Traditional Asian foot massage has enjoyed a big revival in Thailand recently, and most of the salons are staffed by prop-erly trained therapists. It costs less than having a few beers in a bar, and it's therefore a service that most visitors can afford on a daily basis. Even if you're not doing a detox programme, having a traditional Asian foot massage from time to time is a wonderful way to totally relax your body and recharge your batteries, while also cleansing the internal organs, stimulating glandular secretions, and clearing congested energy and nerve channels in the feet.

A convenient way to perform your own deep tissue foot massage is to walk barefoot on smooth round stones embedded in concrete, like little cobblestones. This technique, known as 'treading stones' (*tsai shir-tou*), has been used for thousands of years in China, and also elsewhere in Asia, as a self-healing therapy, and its effects are fast and effective, stimulating points deeply imbedded in the tissues of the feet. You can easily make your own therapeutic stone-walk at home by setting smooth round stones, varying in size from a plum to a peach, halfway into one or two square metres of wet cement, then letting it dry. To use the stones for deep tissue foot massage, walk around slowly on the stones with bare feet, pausing to rock back and forth on your feet whenever you find points that are sore or sensitive. The idea is to soften any hard spots and to dissolve any crystallized particles that you find in your feet by pressing and rubbing those spots on the stones. For best results, you should try to do this for about 20 minutes, twice daily, for a period of one to two weeks. It's also an excellent supplemental therapy for any detox programme, because it greatly accelerates internal cleansing and elimination of wastes, and stimulates healing responses throughout the system.

Nei-dzang *internal organ massage*

TCM also has a special type of massage designed to directly stimulate the internal organs, facilitate their drainage of toxic wastes, and draw circulation of blood and energy into the organs and glands to repair and replenish them. Known as *nei-dzang* (literally, 'internal organ') massage, this technique employs the extended tips of the index, middle and ring fingers to probe deeply into the abdominal cavity and apply massage therapy directly to the internal organs. This direct pressure clears stagnant fluids and disperses congested energy, drives toxic residues from the organ tissues, and stimulates sluggish organs to restore normal function. It's a very effective way to relieve abdominal bloating and water retention, move clogged bowels, clear liver congestion, reduce swelling in the pancreas and eliminate gas. Not many therapists are qualified to practise this method today, and it should only be done by someone properly trained to work in the soft tissues of the abdominal cavity, but if you do manage to find a qualified practitioner, it's well worth arranging a series of treatments as a support for any detox programme.

When internal organ massage is performed by a healer who has mastered the skill of 'emitting energy' through the hands, it's known as *chi nei-dzang*, and the results are even more dramatic. The hands of such healers are known as 'flags of energy' in Chinese, because they can wave healing energy directly into the channels of the ailing organs through their palms and fingertips, producing therapeutic effects in the energy system to amplify the physical therapy provided by tactile pressure.

Hot herbal oil massage

In India, Thailand and Bali, a form of traditional therapeutic massage using hot herbal oils and based on the principles of classical *ayurvedic* medicine is still widely practised. Natural massage oils such as sesame, sweet almond and coconut are infused with aromatic essential oils known for their purifying and healing medicinal properties and then heated to slightly above body temperature. The hot oil is applied liberally to the body with a vigorous massage, driving the volatile medicinal essences deep into the tissues, where they enter the bloodstream and energy meridiens and circulate throughout the system. This type of massage is particularly effective for curing arthritis, rheumatism and any sort of inflammation in the joints and ligaments. It also drains the lymph channels, tones the skin and soothes the nervous system.

Chiropractic

Chiropractic is a remarkably effective medical therapy that developed as a branch of Western medicine during the nineteenth century and became very popular for its non-invasive, deeply healing techniques. Since the advent of modern surgery and allopathic drug therapy, however, conventional Western doctors generally discount chiropractic as some sort of voodoo medicine and rarely recommend it to their patients. But just like Dr Lee's traditional Chinese foot massage therapy, chiropractic is based on sound scientific principles and often produces positive results when all modern medical methods fail. Consquently, the public is beginning to rediscover and utilize this form of treatment, which realigns all of the major joints and bones in the body and rebalances the entire skeletal framework. Misaligned bones, especially in the neck, spine and sacrum, can cramp and obstruct nerve and energy channels, depriving the related organs and glands of energy and blocking nerve signals to them from the brain. By loosening up the joints and ligaments and manipulating the bones back into proper alignment, the free flow of blood, energy, and nerve impulses is restored to all of the internal organs, thereby allowing them to cleanse and heal themselves. During prolonged periods of toxicity, the body stores many toxic wastes as crystalline deposits in the joints, gradually throwing posture off balance and pushing bones out of position. Therefore, a few chiropractic adjustments either before or during a detox programme can assist the body's cleansing and healing mechanisms to function more efficiently.

Self-massage

Self-massage is a simple, convenient technique that may be applied any time, any place to help keep bodily fluids moving, release tension and toxins from tissues, and relieve the minor aches and pains that can arise in the body during the detox process. Anyone can do it, and it requires no special training.

When practising self-massage, it's best to sit on a chair or stool with the spine straight and feet flat on the floor. Before you start, rub the palms of the hands together briskly for about 30 seconds, until they feel warm, in order to charge them with energy and increase their polarity. This enhances the therapeutic benefits of self-massage, especially when working on vital points along the energy meridiens. Recharge the palms in this manner every 2–3 minutes throughout the treatment.

Acupressure

There are several major energy points on the body that may be effectively stimulated for detox purposes by means of self-acupressure. It's important to remain as relaxed as possible while doing this, because energy cannot flow freely through tissues that are 'uptight' with physical tension. It's also best to do this while breathing deeply and slowly from the diaphragm, to help circulate blood and energy and keep the nervous system in the restorative parasympathetic mode.

The four most useful points for self-acupressure during detox, illustrated in Fig. 2, are briefly described below:

Ho-gu ('valley of harmony') This is one of the body's primary power points, and stimulation here gives a boost to the entire energy system. It is located on the large intestine meridien, in the V-shaped depression in the webbing between the base of the thumb and index finger. Press the tip of the thumb deeply into the 'valley' until you find this sensitive point, then push hard on it for about 10 seconds, release, rub the surface in circles, and repeat two or three times. This point stimulates the colon, relieves headaches and toothaches on the side pressed, alleviates fatigue and improves respiration, all of which are benefical to the detox process.

Tai-chung ('supreme thruster') This point is the equivalent on the foot to the 'valley of harmony' point on the hand. Located along the liver meridien on top of the foot, the point is tucked in between the tendons of the big and second toes, about 3 cm up from the slot between those toes. Press the thumb deeply between these two tendons until you find the point, then apply

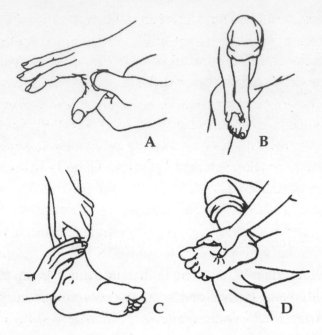

Fig. 2 **Four vital acupressure points for practising self-massage therapy**

pressure in the same way as described above. This is the most
powerful point on the liver meridien, and acupressure here
stimulates all liver functions, prompts liver detoxification, helps
cure hepatitis and other liver disease, relieves headaches and
eyeaches caused by congestion and 'fire' in the liver, and is also
a good way to take the edge off a hangover.

San-yin-jiao ('triple yin intersection') Located at the junction
where the meridiens of the three primary yin organs (liver,
kidneys and spleen) intersect on the inside of the calf, this point
is found one hand-width above the ankle, along the inside edge
of the shin bone. Both the liver and kidneys are primary excretory organs, and pressure on this point provides strong stimulation to both. It also governs sexual energy, enhancing potency
in men and helping to regulate menstrual cycles in women. It's
a good point to press for an energy boost when your vitality is
running low during detox.

Yung-chuan ('bubbling spring') This is the most powerful point on the kidney meridian, located in the centre of the ball of the foot, 5 cm down from the middle toe. Pressure here stimulates kidney functions and energizes the entire system. It is also specifically effective for treating hypertension, anxiety and insomnia, and for balancing irregular heart rhythms. In addition, this point stimulates the adrenal glands, which are attached to the kidneys, to secrete hormones that enhance vitality and help keep the entire endocrine system in balance.

Squeezing (ya) *and rubbing* (mo)

This technique may be applied to the flesh and joints of the neck, shoulders, arms and legs to stimulate drainage of lymph channels, activate blood circulation, drive toxic residues from tissues and release tension from muscles and tendons. Rub the palms together to charge them with energy, then use the fingers and thumb of the right hand to grab and give a strong squeeze to the muscles and tendons on the left side of the body, then briskly rub the surface with the open palm. Start at the neck and shoulder, work down the arm to the fingers, and massage from the top of the thigh down the leg to the toes. Then use the left hand to work on the right side of the body.

'Chi *brushing'*

This method uses the charged palm of the hand as a 'brush' to disperse congested energy from various tissues and organs, thereby opening circulation of blood and energy to those tissues, clearing stagnation and draining toxins. It's also a good way to relieve minor aches in the body. After charging the hands by rubbing them together till warm, use one palm to repeatedly brush in a downward direction across the surface of the tissues you wish to treat, as though you were trying to wipe off something from the skin and sweep it away. For example, if the muscles of your arms or legs ache, brush a charged palm across the aching muscles, always sweeping downward and away from the body. This 'scatters chi' (*san chi*) from tissues where energy and fluids have become congested and stagnant, relieving the pain and reducing the inflammation that such congestion causes. If you wish to clear and soothe an aching liver, use the charged palm of your left hand to reach across and brush down across the surface of the skin directly over the liver. Since this therapy works primarily on the level of energy, the clearing and soothing effects are not solely confined to the physical surface where the brushing is applied; the hand functions as a sort of 'energy wand' to transmit therapeutic benefits deep into the tissues beneath the surface.

While we're on the topic of 'brushing', another tried-and-tested way to facilitate rapid detox by self-massage is by dry-brushing the entire surface of the body, except for the head, using a dry bath brush made with natural plant bristles. Brush briskly down the inside and outside of the arms, from shoulders to hands, down the entire surface of the legs, from hips to feet, and down the front and back of the torso and both sides of the ribcage, moving from the neck down to the waist. This is an excellent way to activate lymph drainage and stimulate micro-circulation of blood in surface tissues. It also strips away dead skin cells and stimulates the generation of new skin, which is a highly beneficial effect during detox.

Tapping (chui-da)

Rhythmically tapping various tissues of the body produces a vibrational wave that carries therapeutic stimulation deep into the body and also penetrates the bone and marrow. Tapping therapy has manifold benefits that assist the detox process. It scatters congested energy and stagnant fluids from surface

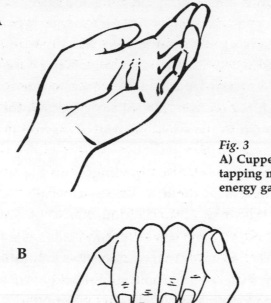

A

Fig. 3
A) Cupped palm for
tapping meridiens and
energy gates

B

B) Clenched fist for tapping
meridiens and energy gates

tissues as well as internal organs, activates blood circulation and lymph drainage, stimulates glandular secretions, clears blocked meridiens, and loosens toxic residues from nerves and other tissues. By virtue of the piezoelectric effect, the vibrations resonate into the crystalline structure of the bones, which transform them into energy pulses that stimulate production of white blood cells and other immune factors in the marrow. This effect strengthens immune response, thereby making the detox process more efficient.

There are two basic ways to apply tapping therapy. One way is to slightly curl the fingers and thumb to form a concave 'cup' in the palm (Fig. 3A). This creates a little 'echo chamber' in the palm that amplifies the tapping vibrations and resonates them within the hollow cavities of the chest and abdomen, where they stimulate the organs and glands. This technique is particularly effective for dislodging toxic residues from the lungs and abdominal organs. First charge the hands, then use the cupped palm of one hand to slap and tap down the opposite side of the ribs from armpit to hip, and from the collarbone down the front of the chest and torso to the waist, then do the same thing with the other hand on the other side.

Another technique is to curl your fingers all the way down to form a fist, with the thumb pressed against the side of the index finger, rather than across the knuckles (Fig. 3B), and to use the curled knuckles and the butt of the palm as a mallet to tap the body. This method is most effective for rattling toxic deposits loose from nerve tissue and stimulating hormone secretions in the endocrine glands. It also has a strong piezoelectric effect on the crystalline structures within the body.

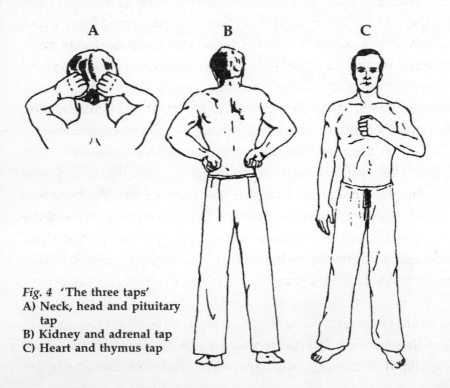

Fig. 4 'The three taps'
A) Neck, head and pituitary
   tap
B) Kidney and adrenal tap
C) Heart and thymus tap

There is also a traditional self-tapping set drawn from *chi gung* practice that may be applied as a highly effective therapeutic support during detox. Known as 'the three taps' (Fig 4), it's an excellent morning exercise to give a daily boost to immune response and balance the endocrine system. I have described it in several of my previous books, but since it's so useful for detox and only takes about 10 minutes, it's worth a brief review again here. It involves the rhythmic tapping of three parts of the body where important glands are located: the head and neck (pituitary), the centre of the chest over the heart (thymus), and the kidneys (adrenals). Spending 3–4 minutes on each one is sufficient to obtain therapeutic benefits. The Three Taps are briefly explained below:

Neck and head tap
Rub the hands together to charge them with energy, then roll the fingers into a fist, with the thumbs pressed against the sides of the index fingers. Use the palm-side of the fists to drum vigorously along both sides of the vertebrae in the neck, alternately left and right, starting at the top of the shoulders and moving slowly up along the neck, continuing up the back of the skull and over the top of the head to the hairline, then drumming back down to the neck again. Tap a bit harder and longer on the area where the neck runs into the base of the skull. The tapping vibrations reverberate through the skull into the head, stimulating hormone secretions from the pituitary gland, dislodging toxins from the tissues of the brain and the thick nerve cords in the neck, and activating circulation of blood and energy in the head. It's a great way to clear 'cobwebs' from your head in the morning and stimulate cerebral functions.

Chest tap
For this exercise, use the second row of knuckles on the fist of one hand to rhythmically rap on the breastbone in the centre

of the chest, directly over the heart. Time the tapping to a beat of one heavy tap followed by two lighter taps: ONE, two three; ONE, two, three, etc. This pattern specifically stimulates the thymus gland, which is located directly beneath the breastbone and whose secretions play a vital role in immune response. One of the first symptoms of AIDS is a radical reduction in the production of immune factors from the thymus gland known as 'T-cells'. Daily tapping on the thymus gradually increases the size of this important gland, which tends to shrink with age, and stimulates secretion of T-cells and other immune factors. This exercise also loosens impacted toxins from lung tissue and has a stimulating effect on the heart.

Kidney tap

To tap the kidneys, use the back of the hands to gently tap the kidneys, alternately left and right, from top to bottom, covering the area on the back from the soft tissue just below the ribcage up to the third rib. The vibrations stimulate secretions in the adrenal glands, which sit like hats on top of the kidneys and whose hormones regulate a wide range of vital functions. Chronic stress depletes the adrenals, so this is a good way to recharge them. As in all three taps, the vibrations work on both the physical level, by vibrating the glandular tissues, and on the energy level, by virtue of the piezoelectric effect on the crystalline structures within the glands. In addition, the kidney tap dislodges toxic deposits in kidney tissues and helps break up crystallized acid wastes before they can form kidney stones. This makes it particularly effective as a kidney support during detox.

Soft exercise

Many people these days completely avoid exercise because they associate it with panting and sweating, strain and injury, toil and trouble. The popular Western notion of exercise includes such heart-racing, joint-grinding, tendon-tearing activities as jogging and weightlifting, tennis and football, surfing and skiing, activities which most people are neither fit nor inclined to do. As a result, when it comes to exercise, the population is divided into a small minority that does it, and an overwhelming majority that just watches.

In Asia, exercise has traditionally been regarded as something one does for therapeutic purposes, not for fun, and it still plays a key role in most traditional Eastern medical systems. Like all 'medicine', the first principle of exercise is that it should 'do no harm'. That obviously eliminates any activity that strains the body, injures tissues and leaves one exhausted. Instead, traditional Asian exercises, particularly Chinese styles, are designed to help the body repair and heal itself, to assist the blood and lymph in detoxifying tissues and excreting wastes, and to energize rather than deplete the system. Such exercises are known as 'soft exercise'. In addition to being soft, they are also very slow and smooth.

In his great masterpiece, *Precious Recipes*, written some 1,500 years ago, the renowned Tang Dynasty physician Sun Ssu-mo states:

> The Tao of nurturing life requires that one keep oneself as fluid and flexible as possible. One should not stay still for too long, nor should one exhaust oneself by trying to perform impossible tasks. One should learn how to exercise from nature by observing the fact that flowing water never stagnates and a busy door with active hinges never rusts or rots. Why? Because they exercise themselves perpetually and are almost always moving.

Let's take a quick look at some of the basic differences between 'hard' Western style exercise and traditional Eastern 'soft' style exercise. Soft exercise focuses on stretching the muscles and tendons and loosening the joints and limbs, thereby opening all the tissues of the body to the free flow of blood and energy. Hard exercise contracts the muscles and compacts the joints, blocking circulation and retaining toxic wastes in the tissues for a long time. Soft exercises are done in conjunction with deep, slow, diaphragmatic breathing, which oxygenates and alkalizes the blood and tissues, while hard exercises force the breath into a shallow, panting mode that utilizes only the narrow upper sections of the lungs. This type of fast shallow breathing in the upper lungs exposes only a very small fraction of the lungs' surface area to incoming air, greatly reducing the intake of oxygen and the discharge of carbon dioxide. As a result, the blood and tissues become increasingly acidic and oxygen-deficient for as long as the exercise continues.

That's not all. Hard exercise causes a rapid accumulation of lactic acid in the tissues, thereby contributing to acidosis. Lactic acid is a metabolic waste produced by muscular exertion, and the last thing you want to do during detox is to produce more acid wastes. By contrast, soft exercise, which requires only minimal muscular exertion, avoids the accumulation of lactic acid in the tissues, and since it is usually done in conjunction with deep breathing, it actually alkalizes and oxygenates the bloodstream, rather than loading it with acids and carbon dioxide. Hard exercise strains the heart by forcing it to race in order to accelerate circulation of blood to the muscles. Furthermore, since hard exercise makes the breath grow shallow, the diaphragm is not engaged in the breathing process, and therefore the heart must bear the full load of pumping extra supplies of blood through the body. Soft exercise combined with deep breathing effectively turns the diaphragm into a 'second heart', engaging it to help pump blood through the circulatory system by virtue of differential pressures in the abdominal and chest cavities. This takes a huge workload off the heart, and when practised daily, the cumulative benefits to the heart can be life-saving.

Perhaps most important, soft exercise performed in conjunction with deep slow breathing shifts the autonomic nervous system into the calm, cleansing, healing mode of the parasympathetic branch and keeps it in this mode. This is an important point because, unless you take effective measures to unwind, relax and keep the parasympathetic branch of the nervous system switched on, and the sympathetic branch turned off, for at least a few days, your body's self-cleansing and healing responses will not be able to function properly, and the detox process cannot proceed. Doing soft exercise and deep breathing for an hour or two each day is a very good way to stay relaxed and keep your nervous system in the healing detox mode.

The best types of soft exercise for detox purposes are stretching and loosening manoeuvres, such as those found in yoga and in the Chinese exercises associated with Tai Chi and *chi gung*. Stretching the muscles squeezes stagnant venous blood out of the tissues, while the subsequent relaxation phase allows fresh arterial blood to flow in. Since these movements are always done softly, slowly and smoothly, with minimal exertion, they do not result in the accumulation of lactic acid in the tissues, they don't race the heart and they don't shorten the breath. Stretching also keeps the nerve and energy channels open and active, and stimulates lymph drainage.

There are many good books on yoga available today, and lots of qualified yoga teachers. As for traditional Chinese stretching and loosening exercises, I have described and illustrated several dozen of these in previous titles (see *The Tao of Health, Sex & Longevity, Guarding the Three Treasures*, and *The Complete Guide to Chi Gung*). Prior to practising these exercises, it's important to familiarize yourself with the basic principles of *chi gung* movement and breathing, and observe a few precautions, which is why I have referred the reader to the books mentioned above for guidance.

If you simply don't like doing repetitive formal exercises, almost any type of gentle, slow activity that does not race the heart or shorten the breath, but that does move the 'water' and activate the 'hinges' of the body, may be done instead as a way of keeping fluids flowing and tissues toned during detox. A long stroll on the beach or a hike in the forest, paddling slowly around in a swimming pool or in the ocean, tending a garden – any such activity will do the trick, as long as you do it softly, slowly and smoothly. If you're a confirmed 'couch potato' and flatly refuse to do even that, then at least you can pay someone else to keep your blood and other bodily fluids moving and your tissues active with therapeutic massage.

The bottom line is this: the blood, the body and the breath are designed to move, not to stand still and stagnate. Anything that remains still and stagnant for too long invariably loses its vitality and starts to decay. So the basic message here is, 'Move it before you lose it!'

CHAPTER 4

Air: The Breath of Life

Most people take a lot of time and trouble each day over the quantity and quality of the food they eat, yet pay only scant attention to drinking sufficient amounts of good water, and take air and breathing entirely for granted. In terms of life's requirements, however, most people have their priorities back to front. As *chi gung* Master Hung Yi-hsiang of Taiwan often reminded his students, 'You can live two months without food and two weeks without water, but you can only live a few minutes without air.'

Air contains essential elements that are at least as important as those derived from food and water as sources of nourishment for life, and proper breathing contributes even more to health and longevity than proper eating. The fact remains, however, that very few people today know how to breathe correctly. Add to that the fact that most of the air in the world has now become as denatured and contaminated with pollutants as food and water, and it becomes clear that most people these days do not take in sufficient supplies of good quality air, depriving their bodies of the essential elements in air that are required to sustain optimum health and vitality. Even when air quality is good, unless you breathe correctly, your body cannot properly assimilate, circulate and utilize the essential elements contained in air, nor can it properly perform a wide range of other vital functions that are directly dependent on correct breathing.

Breath is the bridge that links body and mind. As the only vital autonomous function that can be consciously controlled by the mind, breathing may be utilized as a sort of tuning device to balance and harmonize all of the other functional systems in the body, and as a pump to replenish all the vital organs and tissues with fresh supplies of blood and energy. Thus, by consciously regulating the breath, the mind becomes capable of directly adjusting the conditions and balancing the functions of all the internal organs and glands in the body. Moreover, by correcting imbalances in the human energy system and increasing the supply and flow of energy, breathing exercises manifest therapeutic benefits for the mind as well as for the body, enhancing mental clarity and improving cerebral functions, because body and mind are both dependent on the same basic energy of life.

Fifteen minutes of slow, regulated, deep breathing gives an immediate boost to blood circulation, lowers blood pressure, alkalizes and oxygenates the bloodstream, stimulates glandular secretions, improves digestive functions and activates detox and immune responses throughout the body by switching the nervous system into the healing parasympathetic mode. At the same time, it calms the mind, pacifies the emotions and banishes stress by switching off the 'fight or flight' action circuit of the autonomic nervous system, thereby stopping secretions of stress hormones such as adrenaline and cortisol.

If you doubt the direct connection between the way you breathe and the way you feel emotionally and mentally, then try this: next time you find yourself all wound up in a state of anxiety, stress or anger, pause for a moment and check the condition of your breathing. You'll discover that whenever you feel 'uptight' or 'pissed off' from anxiety or anger, your breath grows very short and shallow and remains lodged high in the upper chest, while the diaphragm remains frozen. Now sit up straight, with your spine erect, and do a few minutes of slow, deep breathing, using the diaphragm to drive and regulate the breath from below and drawing air deep down into the lower lobes of the lungs. Presto! Anxiety and anger evaporate into thin air, body and mind relax and release their tension, and a soothing state of calm flows like a wave through the entire system. A state of anxiety or anger simply cannot be sustained when the breath is consciously kept slow, deep and diaphragmatic, because deep breathing immediately switches the nervous system off the 'fight or flight' action circuit and shuts off the flow of stress hormones and neurotransmitters.

Good air and correct breathing may therefore be utilized as effective therapeutic tools to prevent and cure disease, to assist and accelerate detoxification and regeneration of the body, and to harmonize both body and mind by balancing the entire energy system. In *Precious Recipes*, the centenarian Tang dynasty physician Sun Ssu-mo states:

> When correct breathing is practised, the myriad ailments will not occur. When breathing is depressed or strained, all sorts of diseases will occur. Those who wish to nurture their lives must first learn the correct methods of controlling breath and balancing energy. These breathing methods can cure all ailments great and small.

First let's review the basic principles involved in learning 'the correct methods of controlling breath and balancing energy', and see how these methods may be applied to support the detox process. Then we'll take a closer look at air itself and find out what makes it such an essential element of life, and how it may be used as a supplement to help detoxify and regenerate the body.

The art of breath control

The key to mastering the art of breath control is to actively engage the diaphragm to serve as a pump to drive the breath. If you observe the way an animal or a baby breathes while sleeping, you'll notice that the abdomen expands on inhalation and contracts on exhalation, while the chest itself remains still. That's due to natural diaphragmatic breathing, which is the way our bodies were designed to breathe. Due to sedentary lifestyles, poor physical posture, obesity and the inhibiting effects of chronic stress and fatigue on respiration, adults tend to breathe high up in their chests, using the clavicles and upper ribs to suck air into the narrow spaces at the top of the lungs, rather than using the diaphragm to draw the breath down towards the abdomen and fill the large lower lobes of the lungs with air. Clavicular upper chest breathing, which is extremely inefficient, is an emergency response to anxiety and stress, and it's the mode of breathing associated with the hyperactive 'fight or flight' instinct. For most adults today, this has become their habitual way of breathing.

In proper diaphragmatic breathing, the diaphragm descends downwards into the abdominal cavity on inhalation (Fig. 5A),

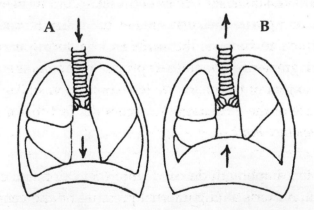

Fig. 5 **Using the diaphragm to drive the breath**
A) Inhalation
B) Exhalation

expanding the lower lungs and allowing them to draw air deep down into the spacious chambers of the lungs' lower lobes. On exhalation (Fig. 5B), the abdominal wall is drawn inwards and the diaphragm rises upwards, driving air out of the lungs in a strong, steady stream. Not only is diaphragmatic breathing the most efficient way to breathe, it also utilizes the diaphragm to perform another vital function for which it was designed: to assist the heart in pumping blood through the body, thereby taking a huge workload off the heart muscle and prolonging the life of the whole organism. Respiratory expert Dr A. Salmanoff describes the cardiovascular functions of the diaphragm as follows:

> It is the most powerful muscle in the body; it acts like a perfect force-pump, compressing the liver, the spleen, the intestines, and stimulating the whole abdominal and portal circulation.
>
> By compressing the lymphatic and blood vessels of the abdomen, the diaphragm aids the venous circulation from the abdomen toward the thorax.
>
> The number of movements of the diaphragm per minute is a quarter of those of the heart. But its haemodynamic power is much greater than that of cardiac contractions because the surface of the force-pump is much greater and because its propelling power is superior to that of the heart. We have only to visualize the surface of the diaphragm to accept the fact that *it acts like another heart*.

When the diaphragm descends into the abdominal cavity on inhalation, it exerts strong internal pressure on the vena cava, a major vein that drains stale blood from the abdominal organs and delivers it up to the heart and lungs to discharge carbon dioxide and replenish the blood with fresh oxygen. The descending diaphragmatic pressure acts like a force-pump to drive stale blood from the internal organs through the vena cava up to the chest. This saves the heart an enormous amount of energy and effectively transforms the diaphragm into a 'second heart' to help drive circulation.

Furthermore, when you consider the fact that the brain is irrigated by about 2,000 litres of blood per day, and that the cerebral cortex contains about 1,000 metres of micro-capillaries per gram, you begin to realize how important it is to keep blood circulating freely through the brain, and what a hard job that is for the heart, a job made even harder by working against the force of gravity. Deep abdominal breathing takes the bulk of this work load off the heart and transfers it to the diaphragm, which helps pump blood up to the brain with each and every breath.

As the diaphragm descends down into the abdominal cavity, it increases internal abdominal pressure, providing a stimulating therapeutic message to all the internal organs and glands, especially the kidneys, adrenal glands and liver, which are sited directly beneath the diaphragm. Listed below are some of the additional health benefits enjoyed by those who practise deep diaphragmatic breathing:

- For every extra millimetre of flex the diaphragm develops on inhalation, lung capacity increases by a volume of 250–300 ml. Studies in China have demonstrated that after six months of breathing practice, the average flex of the diaphragm increases by 4 mm, thereby increasing overall lung capacity by 1,000–1,200 ml per breath.
- A study conducted in India showed that after only 15 minutes of deep diaphragmatic breathing, the average volume of air inhaled per breath rose by 50 per cent, while the average number of breaths per minute dropped from 15 to 5. This makes breathing far more energy efficient and literally 'saves breath'.

- A major study on breathing conducted in China showed a big rise in red blood cell count after only 30 minutes of regulated deep breathing exercise. This greatly enhances the blood's capacity to hold and carry oxygen, which is a major advantage during detox.
- All digestive functions are immediately improved by a session of deep breathing exercise, which stimulates secretions of bile, pepsin and other digestive juices in the liver, stomach and pancreas, and enhances peristaltic contractions throughout the digestive tract.
- Deep diaphragmatic breathing activates the body's innate cleansing and healing responses by switching the nervous system into the restorative parasympathetic branch, thereby triggering the release of neurotransmitters and hormones that signal the body to detoxify and repair itself.

All of these benefits have obvious applications for the detox process and may be easily utilized at any time and in any place during the course of a detox programme to relieve discomfort, assist the detox and healing process, alkalize and oxygenate the blood, eliminate bad moods, relax body and mind, and keep the entire system in an optimum state of internal harmony and balance.

Deep diaphragmatic breathing is performed in four distinct stages, and its therapeutic effects may be further amplified by the three manoeuvres known in *chi gung* and yoga as the 'three locks', which are applied during the retention stage. The four stages are as follows:

Inhalation Relax the diaphragm and let it expand slowly downwards into the abdominal cavity, while drawing in a steady stream of air through flared nostrils and sending it down into the lower lungs. When the lower lungs are full, expand the ribcage and clavicles slightly to allow air in to 'top off' the narrow upper portions of the lungs, then gently press the entire 'bubble' of inhaled air down into the diaphragm, which causes the abdominal wall to bulge out.

Retention Apply the three locks (see below) to 'lock up' the breath and increase the internal pressure within the abdomen and sacrum, retain the breath and hold the locks for 3–10 seconds, no longer, then relax the locks and release the breath.

Exhalation Draw the abdominal wall inwards and let the diaphragm rise upwards into the chest to drive the breath out of the lungs in a long, slow, steady stream of air, either through the nose or through the mouth, depending on the exercise.

Pause Pause briefly after exhalation is complete to allow the abdominal wall and diaphragm to relax again and fall back into place, before commencing the next inhalation.

It is the retention stage that produces the strongest therapeutic benefits in four-stage diaphragmatic breathing, especially when the effects are amplified with the three locks. Retentions of longer than 10 seconds should never be attempted without prior training from a qualified teacher, but even short retentions of 3–10 seconds, which may be safely practised without supervision, provide profound therapeutic effects throughout the body.

Breath retention triggers what's known as the 'dive response', or cellular respiration, whereby heartbeat slows by half and blood pressure drops, while the cells start 'breathing' spontaneously to produce energy by breaking down sugars and releasing oxygen to generate internal body heat. Seals use this mechanism when diving for fish in freezing cold seas, and infants instinctively apply it when submerged underwater, but adults lose it due to incorrect breathing habits. Practising four-stage deep breathing with retention gradually restores this innate metabolic response.

Breathing deeply and briefly retaining the breath instantly calms the nervous system by switching it over to the parasympathetic branch and quickly lowers blood pressure by reducing the pulse. Activating cellular respiration prompts the cells to discharge toxins and produce energy. Breath retention increases the partial pressure of oxygen in the blood against the capillary walls, thereby enhancing the exchange of gas between the blood-stream and the cells. It is also the retention stage of breathing that signals the stomach to secrete pepsin and other digestive enzymes, and stimulates peristalsis in the intestinal tract. In addition, retention applied in conjunction with the three locks squeezes stale blood from the internal organs by increasing abdominal pressure and drives it up through the vena cava to the heart and lungs for replenishment. It also disperses stagnant energy from the organs through the meridien system.

In order to amplify internal pressure within the abdominal cavity and seal it up during the brief retention stage, you may apply the ancient Asian breath enhancement manoeuvres known as the three locks. Here's a quick review of how to do it:

Anal lock

The bottom of the sacral cavity is supported by a web of muscle and sinew known as the 'urogenital diaphragm', which controls the activities of the anus, rectum, bladder, perineum and urogenital canal. As the lungs fill and the diaphragm descends into the abdomen during inhalation, the pelvic floor below is pushed down by growing pressure from the diaphragm above, stretching the tissues of the urogenital diaphragm downwards and reducing internal pressure on the abdominal organs and glands. The downward pressure on the urogenital diaphragm also causes internal energy to leak out through the anal and urogenital orifices.

To prevent this loss of internal pressure and energy, apply the anal lock as soon as inhalation is complete, by deliberately contracting the anal sphincter and extending the contraction to the urogenital orifice, as though you needed to pee and poop but couldn't find a toilet. This tightens all the tissues of the urogenital diaphragm and lifts up the entire pelvic floor. Known in yoga as *mula banda* and in *chi gung* as *ti gang* (literally 'lifting the anus'), the anal lock effectively seals in and prevents the loss of internal pressure and energy from below, thereby helping sustain elevated diaphragmatic pressure within the abdomen and sacrum and amplifying the therapeutic effects of breath retention. Contracting the anus and lifting the pelvic floor at the end of inhalation counteracts the downward push on the urogenital diaphragm and prevents the escape of internal energy and therapeutic pressure from the abdomen and sacrum.

Applying the anal lock flexes the myriad muscles and tendons, nerves and blood vessels of the sacrum, including those involved in urination, bowel movements, orgasm, menstruation and prostate and ovary functions. All of these functions are stimulated and balanced by anal contractions because their tissues are all interwoven within the urogenital diaphragm. Practising this manoeuvre also helps prevent and cure haemorrhoids, by flushing stagnant blood from the clogged capillaries of the anal sphincter and irrigating them with freshly oxygenated blood. In fact, if you carefully observe animals, such as cows and horses, dogs and cats, you will notice that they rhythmically contract and relax the anus a few times immediately after every defecation. This helps propel residual faeces from the rectum at the end of a bowel movement, and replenishes the anal tissues with a fresh circulation of blood and energy.

The anal lock should be held until the end of the retention stage, for 3–10 seconds only, and released at the beginning of exhalation.

Abdominal lock

The abdominal lock is applied immediately after the anal lock is set, by deliberately drawing the abdominal wall slightly inward towards the spine, thereby preventing the loss of internal pressure from the front. As the lungs fill up and the diaphragm descends, the abdominal wall balloons outwards due to growing internal pressure within the abdominal cavity. Unless you pull the abdominal wall back in a bit at the end of inhalation, its outward expansion reduces internal pressure within the abdomen, and some of the therapeutic benefits of retention are lost. Applying the abdominal lock seals internal pressure in from the front, while the anal lock prevents it from escaping below. From above, internal pressure is firmly locked into the abdomen by the descending diaphragm, and the spine provides a strong retaining wall at the back. The abdominal and anal locks thus complete the sealing in of elevated pressure within in the abdomen and sacrum, and the therapeutic benefits of this enhanced internal pressure on the organs and glands continues until the locks are relaxed and the breath released.

Neck lock

The neck lock is not directly involved in maintaining enhanced pressure within the abdomen. Instead, it is designed to help press the breath down into the lower lungs and hold it there, and to prevent enhanced internal pressure in the abdomen from causing a sudden surge of blood to rush up into the brain during the retention phase. The neck lock also pulls on the spinal cord from above, giving it a stimulating stretch. To apply the neck lock, contract the muscles of the throat in the front and close the glottis over the bronchial entrance inside, while also tucking in the chin a bit and slightly stretching up the back of the neck, without bending the neck forward. The neck lock shuts the entrance to the throat, making it much easier to press down and retain the breath, while also partially constricting the carotid arteries to prevent blood from flooding up into the brain. While contracting and closing the throat in the front, the neck lock gives a slight stretch to the neck at the back, opening the nerve and energy channels that enter the head from the spine and giving a therapeutic tug to the entire spinal cord. This stretch activates energy flow in the spinal channels and encourages it to rise up through the meridiens from sacrum to brain, where it energizes all cerebral functions. Partial pressure on the carotid arteries also regulates the heart by slowing and deepening the pulse, greatly increasing cardiovascular efficiency.

Like the other two locks, the neck lock is held until the end of retention, then relaxed with the release of breath at the beginning of exhalation. When applying the neck lock, there is a tendency at first to hunch up the shoulders, which causes tension in the neck and upper back and obstructs the free flow of nerve and energy pulses there, so check your posture after the neck lock is set and make sure your shoulders remain relaxed.

The three locks are applied only when practising complete, four-stage deep breathing exercises in still sitting or still standing postures. When practising moving forms of breathing exercise, such as Tai Chi or the eight pieces of brocade, which involve continuous rhythmic movements of the body, natural two-stage breathing is used, without retention or pause, each inhalation and exhalation following and flowing smoothly into one another in seamless succession, like the swinging pendulums of a clock. Four-stage breathing in still postures and two-stage breathing timed to rhythmic bodily movements each have their respective therapeutic benefits. Four-stage deep breathing with retention is particularly effective for assimilating essential elements from air and discharging toxins from blood and tissues, and for stimulating cellular metabolism. Slow rhythmic body movement synchronized with two-stage deep breathing is best for giving a strong boost to circulation of blood and energy throughout the system, clearing blocked meridiens, transforming stagnant energy, draining lymph channels, and activating all the 'hinges' of the body.

Let's take a brief look at both styles.

Breathing in stillness

Still breathing exercises may be practised either sitting or standing. The traditional standing posture used for practising Chinese breathing exercises is called the 'horse' stance (Fig. 6). Feet should be placed parallel and shoulder-width apart on the floor or ground, with knees slightly bent, pelvis tucked forward, shoulders relaxed and neck straight, arms hanging loosely down with palms facing towards the rear. There should be a straight line running from the crown of the head through the centre of the body to a point midway between the navel and spine, then down through the perineum to a point midway between the feet on the ground. Body weight should rest slightly forward on the

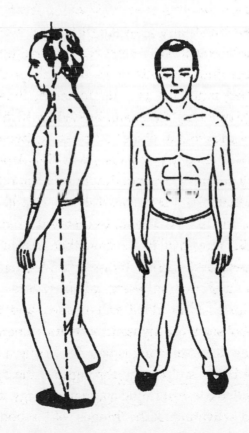

Fig. 6 **The basic horse stance for** *chi gung* **practice**

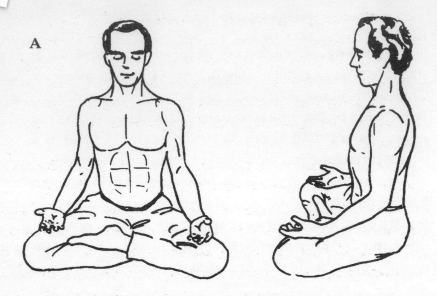

A

Fig. 7. **Two basic sitting postures for still sitting, *chi gung* and meditation: Sitting flat with legs crossed**

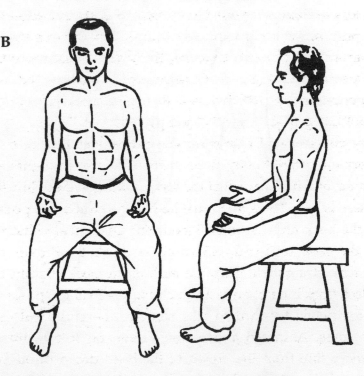

B

Sitting erect on a stool, feet on the floor

balls of the feet, not back on the heels, with the body's centre of balance located in the middle of the lower abdomen, 5 cm below the navel. This point lies in the second chakra, and is known in Chinese as the *dan-tien*, or 'elixir field'. This is the body's 'sweet spot', the place where energy collects when doing breathing exercises and the best place to focus attention while practising deep breathing.

Most people, however, prefer to practise still breathing exercises in the sitting position, which has two basic forms (Fig. 7). One way is to sit with legs crossed on a cushion or mat placed on the floor, either in full- or half-lotus posture. The half-lotus posture, as depicted in the illustration, is much easier to hold for prolonged periods of practice and is therefore recommended for beginners. Alternatively, you may sit on the edge of a low stool or chair, with both feet planted firmly on the floor, parallel and shoulder-width. If sitting crossed-legged on the floor numbs your legs and strains your lower back, you should choose the stool posture, which is very easy to maintain without straining any part of the body. In both forms, the hands should rest relaxed and open on the thighs, with palms up, just above the knees. This permits energy to flow freely through the powerful *lao gung* points located in the centre of the palms.

Regardless of which posture you prefer, standing or sitting, it's very important to pay close attention to proper alignment of the spine; otherwise much of the therapeutic benefit of breathing exercises is lost. The spine must be held as straight as possible, with the neck and sacrum aligned with the spinal column. To align the neck, tuck your chin down towards the throat, at the same time straightening up the back of the neck slightly, as in the Neck Lock but not quite as much as that. To align the sacrum, tuck the pelvis forward to take some of the curve out of the lower spine. As noted above, you should be able to trace an imaginary line from the crown of the head down through the throat and chest to the *dan-tien* point in the centre of the lower abdomen. This is the path of the central channel (also called the thrusting channel), through which the cosmic energies of the sky ('heaven') and the elemental energies in the ground ('earth') travel and mix with the organic energies of the human system ('humanity').

Heaven, earth and humanity (*tien, di, ren*) are known as the 'three powers' in Taoist internal alchemy, and they represent the sum total of all the vital energies in the universe that contribute power to life on earth. Chinese breathing exercises are designed to tap into these infinite sources of primordial energy, and to harmonize and circulate them through the human system to protect health and prolong life. The spine, known as the 'ladder to heaven', links the earth energies that rise up from the ground with the cosmic energies that rain down from the sky, and transforms them into frequencies and patterns that may be utilized by the human energy system. If the spine is blocked or kinked, or misaligned with the head and sacrum, the spinal energy channels cannot properly conduct and transform the various energies which breathing exercises generate.

There are three distinct types of energy that travel through the spine, each within its own respective channels (Fig. 8). The most obvious is nerve signal energy, which travels through the spinal cord and links the brain to the peripheral parts of the body. During deep breathing exercises, the calming parasympathetic branch of the nervous system is activated, linking the brain directly with the endocrine glands that govern detoxification and immune responses. Another form of energy that travels along the spine is the energy that controls the various internal organs. This energy moves through major meridiens located along the spine, which then distribute it to the organs and other tissues of the body through a network of 12 main organ-energy channels and countless smaller branch channels. The third type of energy associated with the spine is the cosmic energy that enters the human system through the crown of the head and

A   B   C

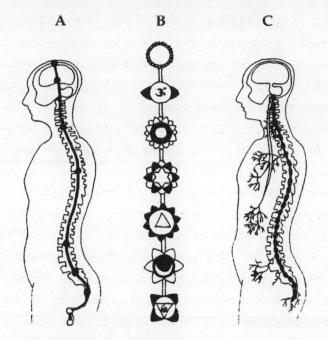

Fig. 8 **Channels, chakras and nerve plexus**
A) The central channel of the meridien network and its major power points
B) The seven 'energy wheels' of the chakra system
**C) The spinal cord and the major nerve plexus of the central nervous
     system**

moves down through the chakra system to the sacrum. The
chakras, known as 'elixir fields' in Chinese, function as energy
transformers to 'step down' the subtle high-frequency energies
that enter the human system from the sky, so that they may be
utilized by the human body and mind. All of these various vital
energies flow first through the main spinal channels, which then
disperse them via branch channels to the organs and tissues. If
the spine is misaligned, cramped or blocked due to injuries or
habitual poor posture, all three forms of energy are obstructed
and become stagnant, and the entire system grows weak and
sluggish and becomes vulnerable to disease and degeneration.

In the yoga tradition of India, deep breathing exercises are
known as *pranayama* and are practised in conjunction with
various yoga postures called *asanas*, or sitting still with legs

crossed. However, *pranayama* should only be practised under the guidance of a qualified teacher, since some of the breathing techniques it employs are quite powerful and complex and, if not performed precisely right and in correct sequence, can cause serious internal energy deviations.

In China, deep breathing exercises are a branch of *chi gung* and are practised in both still and moving modes. *Chi gung*, which literally means 'energy work' or 'breathing skill', is usually practised in synchronized conjunction with slow body movements, but there are also still forms that may be practised standing or sitting. Basic *chi gung* breathing exercises may be safely practised by beginners from a book, without prior instruction from a teacher, as long as the basic guidelines on form and posture are followed, and breath retention never exceeds 10 seconds. I give detailed instructions for a variety of such exercises in several of my previous books, particularly *The Tao of Health, Sex & Longevity*, *Guarding the Three Treasures* and *The Complete Guide to Chi Gung*, so will limit the discussion here to one simple breathing exercise that can be easily practised anywhere and at any time. Called *tu na*, literally 'expel and collect', it facilitates internal cleansing, alkalizes and oxygenates the bloodstream, calms the mind, soothes the nerves, rebalances the entire energy system, and it is both safe and easy to do.

Tu na breathing has been practised in China for thousands of years as a simple and effective means of healing and preventive health care. It involves the four-stage breathing sequence, with the three locks applied during a brief retention. The idea is to first 'expel' stagnant air from the lungs and stagnant energy from the meridiens with a long, strong exhalation, then 'collect' fresh air and energy with a long, deep inhalation. During the retention stage, the bloodstream 'collects' oxygen and negative ion energy from air in the lungs, and the cells in turn 'collect' it from the blood through the capillaries; thus the whole system is completely recharged. In order to ensure balance and stability, *tu na* should be practised in one of the still sitting postures, not standing, at least until the body grows accustomed to the enhanced circulation of blood and energy, after which it may be practised standing in the 'horse' position as well.

Adopt a stable sitting posture, with spine erect and head aligned with sacrum, then flare open the nostrils and commence a long, slow inhalation, drawing the air down deeply into the lower lungs, then 'topping off' the upper lungs and gently sinking the entire breath as far down into the diaphragm as possible. Immediately apply the anal, neck, and abdominal locks, relax the shoulders, and retain the breath for just 3–5 seconds; later you may work up to longer retentions of 5–10 seconds, if you wish. Then relax the locks and release the breath, exhaling in a long, steady stream while gradually drawing in the abdominal wall and letting the diaphragm rise up into the chest cavity to completely expel the breath. Pause briefly and allow the diaphgram and abdominal muscles to relax again, then start the next inhalation. In order to obtain effective therapeutic results, *tu na* should be practised for at least 15 minutes per session.

Exhalation may be done either through the nose or mouth, depending on which aspect of the exercise you wish to emphasize – elimination or assimilation. Exhaling through the nose places primary emphasis on the 'collect' aspect, allowing the blood and tissues to rapidly assimilate and store fresh supplies of oxygen and energy. Exhaling through the mouth shifts the emphasis to the 'expel' phase, increasing the discharge of carbon dioxide from the blood, expelling residual stale air from the lungs, and driving stagnant energy from the meridiens. Both types of exhalation may be practised at the same sitting. There are two ways to exhale through the mouth: one is to purse the lips and blow the breath out in a long steady stream through a narrow slit in the mouth, as though trying to move a candle flame a metre in front of your face without blowing it out; the other is to constrict the top of the throat by partially closing the glottis, then exhaling the breath slowly and strongly from the back of the mouth while making a low, hoarse 'haw' sound.

Another form of this breathing exercise is to combine it with long, rhythmic extensions of the spine, as shown in Fig. 9. To do this, sit on the edge of a stool or chair, with feet planted firmly on the floor and hands placed palms-down on the thighs above the knees. Inhale, apply the three locks, and briefly retain

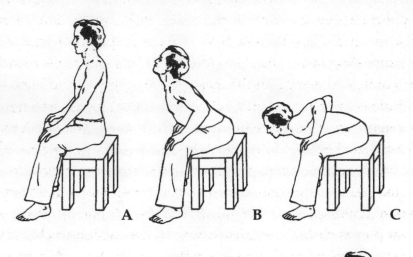

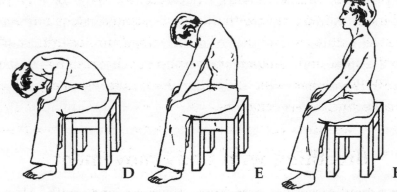

Fig. 9 Tu-na chi gung **breathing with spinal stretch movement**
A) Starting posture; inhale
B) Extend chin and stretch forwards; start exhalation
C) Full stretch forwards; complete exhalation
D) Tuck chin in and arch spine up; breath pause
E) Straighten back up; start inhalation
F) Return to start; complete inhalation

the breath while sitting with spine erect, then relax the locks and jut the chin out in front, extending the spine as you stretch slowly forward and down in synchronicity with exhalation, timing it so that your body is extended fully forward at the end of the exhalation stage. Then relax the neck and let the head hang down naturally for a brief pause, before commencing the next inhalation and returning the spine back to erect position by pushing the body up slowly with the hands pressing on the thighs for support. Apply the three locks again, hold briefly, and start another round. This exercise flexes the entire spinal cord and all its supporting muscles and tendons, and also realigns the spinal vertebrae, stimulating all the major nerve networks and energy meridiens located along the spine, and activating the free flow of cerebrospinal fluids within the spinal shaft. The rhythmic arching and bowing of the spine also activates the seven chakras and stimulates secretions of vital hormones from the respectively related glands – pineal (crown chakra), pituitary ('third eye' chakra), thyroid (throat chakra), thymus (heart chakra), adrenals (solar plexus chakra), testicles/ovaries (lower abdomen chakra), and prostate/vaginal glands (root chakra). A good way to combine still sitting *tu na* with the moving spinal extension form is to start with a few minutes of the moving form to stretch and align the spine and stimulate the nerves and chakras, then finish with 10–15 minutes in the still sitting form to focus on expelling and collecting air and energy.

Breathing with body movement

Deep diaphragmatic breathing synchronized with slow, rhythmic body movements, performed in a state of physical relaxation and mental calm has been practised as a form of preventive and curative health therapy in China since ancient times. As the great Chinese alchemist and healer Ko Hung explained in the 4th century AD, 'The onset of illness is a sign that energy is not flowing. One must exercise in order to unblock the myriad meridiens and facilitate the free flow of energy.'

Synchronized breathing and body movement provides a powerful dynamic boost to the circulation of blood and energy throughout the body. Since these exercises are always practised slowly, softly and smoothly, with minimal muscular exertion, they do not cause a build-up of lactic acid in the tissues, as hard exercise does. Deep diaphragmatic breathing enhances the free flow of blood and energy, driving them through their respective channels, while the long extensions of the limbs and gentle twists and turns of the torso guide this enhanced circulation out to the farthest extremities of the body and into the deepest tissues of the internal organs. This quickly clears the meridiens of stagnant energy and purges the organs and other tissues of stale blood, suffusing every cell in the body with fresh supplies of both. TCM has always viewed the free flow of blood and energy as primary foundations of health, and imbalances in either as the basic causes of disease. The famous physician Hua To, who lived a century before Ko Hung and treated princes and peasants alike, stated this principle very succinctly: 'When the blood pulses unobstructed through the veins, illness cannot take root.'

Hua To developed a series of gentle rhythmic breathing exercises based upon the movements of animals in nature, and prescribed them as curative therapy for a wide range of ailments, including arthritis, rheumatism, digestive difficulties, heart and circulatory problems and nervous system disorders. Known as *dao yin* ('induce and guide'), these exercises induce the flow of blood and energy and guide them as they circulate through the system. Because these forms were based on the way animals move, they were also called *wu chin hsi*, or the 'play of the five creatures'. Cheng Yuan-lin, a contemporary of Hua To, commented on this form of therapy as follows: 'Breathing practised together with the movements resembling a bear, bird and other animals helps move our energy, nourishes our bodies, and builds our spirits.'

This type of therapeutic breathing with synchronized body movement is the basis of all forms of Chinese *chi gung* exercise, which brings body, breath and mind into a unified state of harmony. In Chinese, the ideogram for *chi* may be used to denote 'energy' as well as 'breath' and 'air', reflecting the view that vital energy, not oxygen, is the most essential component in air and that breath is the vehicle for bringing this essential energy into the body. *Gung* refers to any skill or work that takes a long time and lots of practice to perfect. *Chi gung* was originally developed about 5,000 years ago as a sort of therapeutic dance to ward off rheumatism, energy stagnation, respiratory disorders and other ailments caused by the excessively damp climate in the flood-prone plains of the Yellow River valley, where Chinese civilization first evolved. In a text entitled *Dance Verse*, written in the 2nd century AD, the scholar Fu Yi states, '*Chi gung* is an art that pleases the spirit, slows the ageing process, and prolongs life.'

The most widely practised form of moving *chi gung* today is Tai Chi Chuan, the graceful, flowing form of martial art inspired when a Taoist sage observed a snake and crane locked in mortal battle. But Tai Chi is a complex form that requires special training from a qualified master and takes many long years of practice to reach a level of proficiency that delivers concrete therapeutic benefits. Very few people these days are willing to commit the amount of time and effort required to achieve perfection. Fortunately, there are much simpler *chi gung* forms, many of which may easily be learned from a book. These provide equally beneficial therapeutic benefits when practised daily, but take a lot less time and patience to learn to perform properly. These simpler forms include the 'eight pieces of brocade' set, the 'six healing sounds' set, the 'five elements' set and even easier single-step forms.

A brief review of some of the major health benefits provided by regular *chi gung* practice is in order here, so that readers may understand why millions of Chinese people have practised it continuously for thousands of years, and why it's such a suitable system of therapeutic exercise for people today. About three hundred years ago, the Taoist adept Shen Chia-shu, remarked, 'Breathing and related exercises are one hundred times more effective as medical therapy than any drug. This knowledge is indispensable to man, and every physician should study it thoroughly.' The leading edge of modern medical science is finally awakening to the truth of this statement, which has been verified with concrete scientific evidence. Here are some of the facts:

Blood and marrow

Red blood cells, which deliver oxygen to the cells, and one type of white blood cell essential for immune response, are produced in the marrow of bones. Healthy marrow produces 480,000,000 red blood cells per minute. In *The Root of Chinese Chi Kung*, contemporary *chi gung* master Dr Yang Jwing-ming, explains the significance of this as follows:

> According to Chinese medicine, your body deteriorates mainly because your blood loses its ability to feed and protect your body. Your bone marrow produces the red blood cells and one type of the white blood cells, but as you grow older, the marrow . . . produces fewer and fewer useful blood cells . . . . To keep marrow fresh and alive and functioning properly, *chi* must be plentiful and continuously supplied. Whenever there is a shortage of *chi*, the marrow will not function properly.

The best way to ensure a continuous supply of fresh *chi* to the marrow is to practise *chi gung* on a regular basis. During a detox programme, sufficient production of red blood cells is even more important than usual, because the bloodstream requires a very high red blood cell count to supply the additional amounts of oxygen the cells need during detox, and extra white blood cells are needed to keep immune response strong.

Brain and central nervous system
As we have already seen, deep breathing synchronized with slow body movements switches the autonomic nervous system over to the calming parasympathetic branch which governs the body's natural self-cleansing and healing responses. During detox, it's essential to keep your nervous system at rest in this healing mode throughout the programme, and there's no better way to do that than by practising *chi gung* every day.

Electroencephalographic (EEG) devices have shown that *chi gung* energizes and activates the 90 per cent of the brain that in most people lies perpetually dormant. We've all been told that on average we use less than 10 per cent of the more than 15 billion brain cells in our heads, but after a session of *chi gung* the entire brain is brought 'on-line', whether you are consciously aware of it or not. This significantly improves all cerebral functions such as memory and learning, and, in some cases, when diligently practised, it also awakens some of the more extraordinary mental powers which lie dormant in our brains, such as telepathy, ESP, clairvoyance, and so forth. Even more importantly, EEG scans of elderly adults in China who practise *chi gung* daily show a pattern and frequency of brain waves that are normally found only in young children, indicating that those who practise *chi gung* can restore their cerebral functions to those of their youth. Chinese medical literature abounds with references to the *huan tung* ('youth restoring') benefits of *chi gung* practice, and studies using modern EEG technology shed scientific authenticity on this claim.

Chi gung not only charges the brain with energy, it also increases supplies of 'vital essence' by stimulating secretions of important neurotransmitters such as serotonin, dopamine and enkephalins. This effect balances all brain functions, enhances mental clarity and facilitates communications between the brain and peripheral nervous system.

Immune response

We've already seen how *chi gung* enhances immune response by switching the nervous system to the parasympathetic healing mode and by stimulating production of red and white blood cells in the marrow. But it also boosts immunity in several other ways. *Chi gung* stimulates the thymus and other glands to secrete the full spectrum of immune factors, while at the same time inhibiting secretions of the adrenal stress hormones released by the 'fight or flight' response, which have strong immuno-suppressive effects. *Chi gung* also increases production of natural steroids, thereby relieving arthritis without the need to resort to the toxic synthetic steroids which most doctors prescribe for this condition.

One of the most significant recent discoveries about *chi gung* is the fact that it activates the PNI response, or psychoneuro-immunology. PNI is one of the body's most powerful healing mechanisms, whereby specific neurotransmitters secreted in the brain communicate directly with the glands of the immune system to activate detox and healing responses throughout the body. In an article by Kathy Keaton, editor of *Omni* magazine, written in May 1992, she describes this response as follows:

> It's been discovered . . . that there are nerve fibres in the thymus, the immune system's master gland, as well as in the spleen, the lymph nodes and the bone marrow – all vital parts of the immune system . . . . In other words, there's a growing body of evidence to suggest that the brain talks directly to the immune system via this electrochemical version of AT&T [telephone exchange].

In order for the brain to release the neuropeptides that activate the body's glandular immune responses, the mind must remain calm, the body relaxed and the nervous system switched over to the parasympathetic branch. *Chi gung* produces this balanced state of mental calm and physical relaxation quickly and efficiently, providing a convenient tool to activate the PNI healing response and open a direct line of healing biofeedback between the nervous and endocrine systems.

Heart and circulatory system
As we've already noted above, correct breathing transforms the diaphragm into a virtual 'second heart' to assist in the circulation of blood. Studies in China show that 20 minutes of *chi gung* practice reduces the pulse by an average 15 per cent, while increasing overall volume of blood circulated, and that this effect continues for several hours afterwards. This enhancement in circulatory power is due entirely to the way *chi gung* shifts the major burden of work in blood circulation from the heart over to the diaphragm. High blood pressure, which has become a major life-threatening condition throughout the world, can easily be controlled by daily *chi gung* practice, without the need for drugs. A study conducted on 100 cases of chronic high blood pressure and hypertension at the Shanghai Research Institute for Hypertension demonstrated that after only 5 minutes of practice, blood pressure levels in all of the patients began to drop dramatically, and that after 20 minutes their blood pressure fell to the level it normally reached 3 hours after taking the blood pressure drugs prescribed for this condition by modern Western medicine. Ninety-seven of these patients remained permanently free of high blood pressure and no longer needed to use the drugs, simply by continuing to practise *chi gung* at home every day, while the three who declined to continue their practice soon suffered relapses and had to go back on drug therapy.

Digestion

Indigestion has become such a common condition for people on modern Western diets that gastric distress is almost taken for granted as an inevitable side-effect of eating. More than half of all Americans surveyed complain of chronic gastrointestinal discomfort, including gas, bloating, constipation, acid reflux and stomachaches. Studies in China have shown that 15 minutes of *chi gung* practice produces a major elevation in secretions of pepsin and other digestive enzymes in the stomach, and of lysozyme in the salivary glands of the mouth. *Chi gung* balances pH in the stomach, thereby helping prevent 'acid indigestion', and the downward movement of the diaphragm in *chi gung* breathing provides an invigorating massage to the liver, stomach, pancreas and other digestive organs and glands within the abdomen, expelling gas, moving stagnant fluids and stimulating digestive functions.

pH Balance

Acidosis has become one of the great banes of modern life. Excessive acidity of blood and tissues is one of the primary preconditions for the onset of all disease and degenerative conditions; conversely, alkalization of blood and tissues is a primary strategy in healing, and one of the main goals in any detox programme. *Chi gung* quickly alkalizes the bloodstream, thereby restoring proper pH balance so that the blood can flush acid wastes from the cells and tissues. This helps detoxify the body and immediately raises resistance to disease. As Drs Peschier and Michel remarked after conducting extensive studies on the benefits of deep breathing in France:

> Every organic or functional disorder leading to conditions of illness is susceptible to the influence, if not always the cure, of controlled breathing. Controlled breathing is the most outstanding method known to

us for increasing organic resistance . . . . It confers on the balance of the acid/base a regularity which is reestablished with every breath.

Antioxidant effect:
Free radicals are the main culprits in the premature ageing and degeneration of the human body, and antioxidants, also known as 'free radical scavengers', are the body's primary line of defence against free radical damage. Most health enthusiasts are already familiar with antioxidant supplements such as vitamins C and E, the minerals selenium and zinc, and various herbs, but are probably unaware that deep breathing exercises can also greatly enhance the body's antioxidant activity. The most potent free radical scavenger produced in the body is the enzyme superoxide dismutase (SOD). Laboratory analysis of blood samples taken from elderly practitioners of *chi gung* show that after a 30-minute session the level of SOD in their blood rises to more than double the average found in those who do not practise this form of exercise. This finding is particularly significant for detox programmes, because during detox the body requires abundant and continuous supplies of SOD and other antioxidant enzymes to deal with all the free radical activity from the toxins released in the tissues. *Chi gung* is therefore a quick and easy way to double the availability of SOD during a detox programme – as well as in daily life.

For further details about the manifold benefits of *chi gung* for human health and longevity, and for detox in particular, the reader may refer to my previous title, *The Complete Guide to Chi Gung*. The points discussed above suffice to demonstrate how useful *chi gung* can be as a therapeutic tool for human health and healing. The many advantages of *chi gung* as a form of medical therapy include the fact that it costs nothing and is easy to administer; it's safe and effective and has no negative side effects when properly practised; it can be practised at any time and in any place without any special equipment; virtually anyone, including children and the elderly, can learn how to do it; it balances body as well as mind simultaneously to correct problems on both levels; and, best of all, it's 'one hundred times more effective as medical therapy than any drug'.

'Yin particles'

While we all know that we need to breathe air in order to supply our blood and tissues with life-sustaining oxygen, few people realize that there is a lot more to air than just oxygen. What counts most in air quality is not its oxygen content, but rather a particular form of energy that activates healthy air and gives it the dynamic vitality required to sustain life. The source of this essential airborne energy is highly active molecular particles called 'negative ions', each of which has a negative charge equivalent to that of one free electron. In Chinese, these units of negatively-charged energy are called *yin li dze*, or '*yin* particles'. In the Taoist principle of *yin/yang* polarity, *yin* is always the 'negative' pole and *yang* is the 'positive'.

Negative ion count is the most accurate measure of air quality in terms of its benefits for human health. Negative ions are produced in air by the action of wind and sun, especially at high altitudes, and by the movement of air over large bodies of water. That's why since time immemorial people have always felt refreshed and rejuvenated after spending a day at the beach or trekking in high mountains: every breath you take in air that's rich in negative ions recharges your blood and cellular batteries with fresh supplies of purifying, energizing negative ions. All air pollutants, such as smoke, dust and toxic chemicals, take the form of large, sluggish molecules with a positive charge. In urban areas, where the air is especially dense with pollutants, the heavy positive ions slow down and trap the vibrant negative ions in the air, reducing their activity, negating their energy and robbing the air of its vitality and healing potential. Clean country air, for example, contains an average ratio of three negative ions to one positive, while polluted city air has about 500 positive molecules for every negative ion, a massive 1,500-fold drop in air quality. Negative ions are also removed from air by air-conditioning and central heating, severely degrading air quality in modern office and apartment buildings. That's why people who work at desk jobs in air-conditioned offices with sealed windows feel more depleted and 'wiped out' after a day of doing nothing but 'pushing papers' and taking phone calls, than farmers and outdoor construction workers who work up a sweat doing hard physical labour in the sun and open air.

Let's take a look at the negative ion count in the various types of air typically found on the earth today:

Polluted air such as that in factories, airtight urban spaces, chemical plants and heavy traffic, produces 20–200 negative ions/cubic cm/sec. Breathing this sort of air causes illness, stress reactions and toxaemia of the blood and tissues.

Unhealthy air such as that in inner cities, high-rise office buildings and shopping malls, produces 200–500 negative ions/cubic cm/sec. Breathing this grade air can cause headaches, irritability, chronic fatigue and various respiratory problems such as asthma.

Average air such as that in suburbs and lowland farm areas, produces 500–1,000 negative ions/cubic cm/sec. This type of air does not cause any specific health problems, but it also has no positive benefits for health, other than providing basic oxygen requirements.

Good air such as that by the ocean, in a big forest, or in low to medium mountain regions, produces 1,000–2,000 negative ion/cubic cm/sec. Breathing air of this quality has distinctive rejuvenating effects and energizes the whole system. It also helps purify the bloodstream.

Healthy air such as that on high mountains, produces over 4,000

negative ions/cubic cm/sec. This is the purest, most therapeutically beneficial air on earth. It has potent detoxifying properties,
invigorates the blood, recharges the human energy system, and
accelerates new cell and tissue growth. It also stimulates the
brain and activates dormant cerebral powers, which is why the
yogins and hermits of ancient India, China and Tibet often chose
to live in remote caves among the wild and windswept peaks
of Asia's highest mountain ranges. The ancient Chinese ideogram for 'immortal sage' is *hsien*, which consists of the symbols
for 'man' and 'mountain'.

In order to remain healthy and strong, the human body needs
to breathe air with a count of about 2,000 negative ions/cubic
cm/sec. That's the sort of air found at unpolluted seashores,
deep in pristine forests and high up in the mountains. However,
most people today live nowhere near such places, which means
that they are breathing air that's not only half as rich in oxygen
as it was 200 years ago, but that's also critically deficient in the
essential energy of negative ions. The only viable way to compensate for the continuing degradation in air quality throughout the
world today is to increase the efficiency of our breathing
methods.

It's no accident that health resorts and spas have traditionally
been located high up in the mountains, or else along the shores
of oceans and lakes. Long experience has taught us that the air
in the mountains and by the sea has a potent vitality that rapidly
cleanses the bloodstream, energizes the nervous system and
regenerates the body. That vitality comes from the high negative ion count in the air at such locations.

One reason that negative ions are such an important factor in
air, especially for purposes of detox and healing, is that they
function as powerful antioxidants to scavenge free radicals in
the blood and tissues. Considering how toxic most people are
these days, and how polluted the environment, this protective
factor in air is more important than ever for those who wish to

live long in good health. Besides scavenging free radicals, negative ions help eliminate all sorts of other toxins as well, by binding with their positive charge and allowing them to be carried away for excretion.

Air that is rich in negative ions continuously purges tissues of toxins and purifies the bloodstream with each and every breath. During detox, when the blood must carry an overload of toxic wastes from the tissues to the excretory organs for elimination, negative ions become an important ally, because they help keep the bloodstream clean, thereby facilitating the blood's capacity to continuously flush toxins and acid wastes from the internal organs and tissues and deliver them to the excretory drains. Negative ion energy from air also increases the electrical potential of each and every cell in the body, and collectively this boost amplifies the power and vibrance of the entire human energy field. Not only does this increase the body's overall resistance to disease, it also helps shield the body from invasion by aberrant external energies such as those produced by artificial electromagnetic fields, microwaves, atomic radiation and other forms of 'energy pollution'.

The most convenient and effective way to increase your assimilation of negative ions is to practise deep breathing exercises in good quality air on a daily basis. The fact remains, however, that most people are unwilling to take the time and effort required to learn and practise *chi gung*. For such individuals, modern technology has come up with some electronic devices that effectively recharge the air in a room, office or car with high concentrations of negative ions, so that people may assimilate abundant amounts of this essential energy, even while lounging in a hammock or armchair.

One such device is the negative ion generator, which emits a constant stream of negative ions into the air from electrically charged metallic pins. These devices, which come in a variety of sizes and output capacities, may be placed in any office, bedroom, work space or other human habitat, to compensate for negative ion deficiency in the air. Many modern office buildings and high-rise hotels and apartment blocks in Japan are routinely equipped with negative ion generators to purify and energize the air that people must breathe inside, and perhaps this helps account, at least in part, for the fact that the Japanese people continue to lead the world in longevity. There are also special units designed for use in cars, and compact battery-operated units that may be taken anywhere, including on aeroplanes.

The commercial airline industry has for years resisted the call to install negative ion generators on all flights, apparently because doing so would acknowledge that there's been a basic problem with the air on aeroplanes all along. This problem became even worse in the jet age, when the commercial airline industry decided to stop drawing fresh air into aircraft in order to save the costs of pressurizing and heating it at such high altitudes. Instead, the air on all commercial airliners is now re-cycled throughout the duration of all flights, forcing passengers to breathe and re-breathe the same stale, germ-ridden air exhaled by other passengers. On long flights, this situation can pose serious health hazards for unsuspecting passengers, especially those with weak immune systems.

The need for negative ion generators in aircraft was first discovered during the early days of the space programme, when it was noted that early astronauts such as John Glenn could not remain aloft in space for more than one day without experiencing debilitating fatigue and mental confusion. It was the Russians who first recognized that the source of the problem was negative ion deficiency, and they solved it by installing negative ion generators in their spacecraft, which immediately enabled their cosmonauts to endure much longer space flights.

Today, airline passengers throughout the world are complaining of circulatory problems, jet lag, virulent diseases contracted in-flight, breathing difficulties and other health problems, all of which are due primarily to the critical deficiency of negative ions in the air within aircraft. A negative ion generator of sufficient output to infuse a large room with life-sustaining negative ions draws less power than that required by a 60-watt lightbulb, so expense is certainly no excuse for not installing these devices on all aeroplanes. Nevertheless, until the airline industry is compelled by public demand to make the air in aircraft safe and suitable for human consumption by installing negative ion generators (or offering passengers portable units at the beginning of all flights, as they offer earphones for in-flight entertainment), the best way to protect yourself from the dangers of the dead, contaminated air that you're forced to breathe on airline flights is to bring along your own portable, battery-operated negative ion generator. Such units are now available.

During a detox programme, it's very helpful to keep a negative ion generator going in your bedroom while sleeping at night. Not only does this neutralize and precipitate all dust, smoke and other pollutants in the air of the room in which you sleep, it also provides strong, continuous antioxidant activity in your blood and tissues while you're sleeping, so that the detox process may continue efficiently and without interruption even while you're asleep. In addition, it protects you from bacterial infections: the natural decay rate for bacteria in ordinary air today is about 23 per cent, but when air is charged with negative ions, the bacterial decay rate rises more than threefold to 78 per cent. In light of how many patients contract deadly bacterial infections in hospitals today, installing negative ion generators in all hospital rooms would save a lot of lives at negligible expense.

Activated air

A new device – one of the most effective electronic detox technologies on the market today – has recently appeared in Australia. Known as an Activated Air System and manufactured by GEOMED Biomedicine, it generates a stream of air with a negative ion count of 5 million ions/cubic cm/sec and shows great promise as a swift, powerful, totally safe therapeutic tool for treating a wide range of ailments and degenerative conditions caused by blood and tissue toxicity.

The GEOMED Activated Air System works by producing a steady stream of highly ionized air containing the same natural ratios of oxygen and nitrogen as ordinary air. Ionized oxygen greatly improves the blood's capacity to cleanse and nourish the tissues. However, nitrogen is equally important for detox purposes, because it functions as a bonding molecule for the discharge of various waste products, such as uric acid and ammonia. The GEOMED generates both ionized oxygen and nitrogen, thereby producing air that has extremely potent detoxifying and rejuvenating properties.

Inhaling this activated ionized air for a period of just 30 minutes produces an immediate, measurable increase in the body's overall metabolic rate and a huge boost to immune response, particularly antioxidant activity. These effects greatly amplify and accelerate the detox process and facilitate healing and regeneration on the cellular level. Those interested in ordering or obtaining further information about the GEOMED Activated Air System, should contact the appropriate supplier listed in Appendix 2.

'The nose knows!'

While the lungs are designed to assimilate oxygen and discharge carbon dioxide through breathing, the more subtle energy elements in air, such as negative ions and the medicinal energies in the volatile vapours released into the air by aromatherapy, are absorbed primarily by special receptors located in the lining of the nasal passages and sinus cavities. That's why the yogins of ancient India developed the Neti nasal douche (see page 51)

– to keep their nasal receptors clean and sensitive so that the essential energies carried in the air may be freely assimilated. These receptors, when clean and functioning properly, transmit the energy of negative ions and volatile aromatic vapours directly into the energy meridiens, blood vessels and nerves of the head, from where they are distributed to the brain and body.

Aromatic vapours released into the air from essential oils and flowers by evaporation carry the essential energies of those plants and transport their potent therapeutic properties directly into the human system via the nasal and sinus receptors. Medieval Arab physicians frequently noted the fact that when cholera, smallpox and other contagious plagues periodically swept through the Middle East, perfumers and incense makers, who worked daily with the potent aromatic essence of plants, rarely succumbed to these deadly diseases. That's because they were protected by the potent medicinal properties of the natural aromatic plants from which they extracted essential scents. Today, the same phenomenon is observed in professional florists, who work amidst the fragrant energies of fresh flowers and consequently rarely catch colds, the flu or other contagious ailments that routinely infect others.

It should be noted, however, that only scents derived from natural plant sources provide medicinal benefits and may therefore be effectively used for aromatherapy. These include various flowers, seeds, roots, barks, leaves and other plant parts which contain volatile aromatic elements. Synthetic scents have a 'smell', but they don't have any bioactive energies with therapeutic properties, and any well trained nose can instantly detect the difference between natural and synthetic scents, not so much by their actual smell but by the subtle effects of their vibrant energy. Those distinctive effects are produced by the ionized energies released into the air from the essential oils of aromatic plants by the process of evaporation. In Taoist terminology, synthetic substances are devoid of the natural 'essence' (*jing*) required to produce the bio-active 'energy' (*chi*) found in the ionized vapours of medicinal plants. The French medical scientist Dr J. Valent, writing in the journal *L'Hopital* in 1960, explains how aromatherapy works:

> Carried by the bloodstream, the ionized plant aroma impregnates every corner of the body, powerfully revitalizes the polarized and discharged cells, replenishes electronic shortages by recharging the bioelectromagnetic batteries, and disperses cellular residue by dissolving the viscous and diseased substances of body fluids. It oxidizes poisonous metabolic waste products, increases energy balance, frees the mechanism of organic oxidation and of self-regulation, and reaches the lungs and kidneys, whence it is excreted or exhaled without a trace.

Here we see how useful aromatherapy can be when applied to the detox process. The ionized essential energy assimilated from the inhaled vapours of medicinal plants penetrates the deepest tissues of the body and reaches into each and every cell, where it 'disperses cellular residue by dissolving the viscous and diseased substances of body fluids' and 'oxidizes poisonous metabolic waste products', sending them all to the lungs and kidneys for excretion. The practical applications of aromatherapy for detox are obvious: by keeping an aromatherapy vaporizer operating in the rooms in which you sleep at night and spend the most time by day, you saturate the air you breathe with the potent ionized energies of medicinal plants, which enter your system with each and every breath to assist and accelerate the detoxification and healing process.

During the day, you should select essential oils that are known for their strong blood and tissue cleansing properties, such as sage, rosemary and juniper. At night, it's best to use aromas with calming nervine properties, such as lavender, frankincense or sandalwood, to help you sleep well. These also have detoxifying properties, but they are gentler than those used by day, so they won't interfere with your rest.

'Silence is golden'

We've all heard this slogan before, but what does it actually mean? Let's hear what Master Chang San-feng, the Taoist sage credited with developing Tai Chi Chuan 600 years ago, had to say about it. He advised, 'Forget about words and your energy won't scatter.' The Taoist adept and commentator Liu I-ming, writing about 200 years ago, said basically the same thing: 'When the mouth speaks, energy scatters.' And in Tibetan Buddhist tradition, the word for 'speech' is often used to denote 'energy', because speech expends and dissipates a tremendous amount of breath and energy. The only sort of 'speech' that focuses rather than scatters energy is mantra, prayer and harmonious song.

Today, with all the manifold pressures and chronic stress of modern life, many people seem to have acquired a 'motor mouth' syndrome. They feel compelled to sustain a constant stream of small talk, gossip and marathon monologues, regardless of whether or not anyone else is really listening to them. Indeed, some people are so addicted to 'blowing off steam' this way that they talk to themselves constantly, even when there's no one else around to listen. This is not the place to speculate on the psychological and emotional implications of the modern motor mouth syndrome, but it is certainly appropriate to point out here the fact that constant chatter drains away vital energy and depletes your 'bio-batteries'. Since energy is the fundamental fuel required to detox, repair and rebalance the human body, especially during an intensive detox programme, it doesn't make much sense to needlessly waste this vital resource by spewing it out of your mouth in a fountain of words. Far better to remain silent and focus your energy inwards for healing purposes.

It is therefore advisable to speak no more than necessary during a detox programme and to remain as silent as possible, in order conserve your limited supplies of vital energy for internal cleansing. Try to resist spending a lot of time on the telephone talking to friends, or making calls to check on your business affairs; all that can wait until the programme is over. And also try not to spend all afternoon scattering your energy to the wind by gossiping with other guests at spas and health resorts; that definitely slows down the detox process and prevents the nervous system from remaining at rest in the healing mode. Instead, have a massage or steam bath, take a stroll in the forest or along the beach, or practise some *chi gung*. Speak only when necessary to communicate something important, and say it softly, with a minimum waste of energy. By 'saving your breath' this way, you'll also be saving your energy for internal cleansing and healing purposes, and that extra reserve of energy is 'as good as gold' in terms of its value to human health and healing.

And that's why 'silence is golden'.

CHAPTER 5

Food: Detox Diet and Supplements

What you don't eat is actually more important than what you do eat during a detox programme. In fact, the best detox diet of all is to eat nothing. The basic dietary strategy for detox is to totally eliminate all acid-forming foods and beverages and to consume only small amounts of a few simple alkalizing items that provide the mix of essential nutrients required by the body when it's in detox mode. By keeping the diet as simple and sparse as possible, digestive wastes are reduced to a bare minimum, and the enormous amount of energy and enzymes that our bodies normally burn up to meet the constant, complex digestive demands of our daily diets are diverted instead to detox duty. The less food you eat and the more water you drink, the faster and more efficiently your body detoxifies and repairs itself.

On the other hand, some nutrients actively assist the detox process, so whatever you choose to eat during a detox programme should be selected to provide precisely those elements. The most important nutritional elements the body needs in order to purify the bloodstream and detoxify the tissues are enzymes, minerals and trace elements, and vitamins. Animal protein, fat and refined sugar and starch, which constitute about 90 per cent of the calories most people in the West consume these days, are not only useless for detox purposes, they actually block the cleansing process and produce large amounts of acid wastes and putrefactive sludge, and should therefore be strictly eliminated from a detox diet.

Short of fasting, which remains by far the best way to detoxify the body, the dietary approach to detox includes four basic strategies. The first and most important step is to abstain entirely from eating or drinking anything that acidifies the blood and tissues. The next step is to design a detox diet based on just a few simple, unrefined plant-source foods that alkalize the blood and tissues while also providing the basic nutrients the body needs to support the detox process from start to finish. The third step is to select a variety of special supplements made entirely from natural sources to assist and accelerate detox by providing pure, concentrated forms of essential nutrients and alkalizing agents. The fourth step is to reduce calorie intake as much as possible, in order to decrease production of digestive and metabolic wastes and conserve energy and enzymes for detox rather than digestive purposes.

Acid abstinence

'The longest journey begins with a single step.' The first step in the direction of detox is to abstain completely from eating or drinking anything that produces an acid reaction in the digestive tract and leaves acid residues in the blood and tissues. This step should be taken a week or more before you start your full detox programme. Some processed foods, such as refined sugar and starch, as well as many chemical food additives, have addictive properties similar to drugs when consumed in large amounts over long periods of time, and it's much easier on the body to withdraw these items from the diet gradually, rather than stopping their intake suddenly. Switching abruptly from a highly acidic state of toxaemia to an alkaline state of intensive detox can produce the unpleasant withdrawal symptoms popularly known as 'cold turkey'. By starting to abstain from all acid-forming food and drink a week or more before implementing the main parts of your detox programme, you give your body a chance to adjust incrementally to the rigours of the alkalization and detoxification process.

First and foremost, you should eliminate *all* animal-source food products from your diet during detox, including meat, eggs and dairy products. All animal products are extremely acidifying to the digestive tract and bloodstream, and they also produce highly putrefactive protein wastes in the bowels. Cancer cells thrive on animal proteins and multiply rapidly in the highly acidic environment they create in the body, while worms and parasites flourish in the toxic sludge they leave glued to the bowel wall. By eliminating all acid-forming animal products from your diet and taking additional measures to alkalize your blood and tissues, you starve any cancer cells that may be developing in the body and rob them of the acidic environment they require to multiply and form tumours. In light of the pandemic spread of cancer throughout all segments of society today, this preventive strategy against cancer is a primary goal of any detox programme.

Animal-based foods require a tremendous amount of energy and enzyme power to digest and process, far more than plant-based foods. If you eat meat, eggs and dairy products while trying to detoxify your blood and tissues, there is simply no way your body can muster the extra reserves of energy and enzymes it needs to cleanse and repair itself. Rather than using these reserves for detox functions such as dissolving developing tumours, dismantling damaged cells and destroying dangerous microbes, your body will instead be forced to divert most of its energy and enzyme power to digestive duty, in order to process the complex proteins and heavy fats in animal foods, and to deal with the putrid acid wastes they produce in the digestive tract.

This defeats the very purpose of detox and should therefore be strictly avoided.

Another category of food that should be deleted completely from the diet during detox is refined starch, especially white flour products such as bread, pasta, cakes and pastries. These items are highly acid-forming and burn up a tremendous amount of energy and enzymes to process. Moreover, since they provide absolutely nothing of nutritional value to the detox process, they should anyway be cut from the detox diet. All highly refined food products that enter the human body, because they are stripped naked of their essential nutrients, must borrow these missing nutrients from the body's reserves to complete their nutritional profiles, in order that they may be properly digested and metabolized in the body. Consequently, eating highly refined processed foods actually robs the body of the essential nutrients it needs to support the detox process.

The most hazardous dietary item of all in terms of its acid-forming, nutrient-robbing properties is refined white sugar. Refined sugar, or 'sucrose', acidifies the bloodstream faster and more severely than any other food on earth, and by far the worst offender in this category is the sugary sweet, fizzy 'acid bomb' known as the 'soft drink'. One 350-ml serving of Coke, Pepsi or similar soft drink delivers a sugar fix equivalent to about 9 teaspoons of refined white sugar straight to the bloodstream, instantly acidifying the bloodstream to the extreme point that, without an immediate emergency response from the body, it would kill you in a matter of minutes. To counteract the sudden radical rise in blood acidity that a glass of sweet carbonated cola causes, and to re-establish a viable balance in blood pH before you drop dead, you'd have to quickly drink 32 glasses of alkaline water. Of course, nobody drinks 32 glasses of alkaline water after each serving of a soft drink, so instead, in order to prevent death by acidosis, the body reacts swiftly by drawing huge amounts of organic calcium from the bones and teeth and pouring it into the bloodstream to neutralize the excess acids and quickly restore alkaline balance. Calcium is the body's most potent alkalizing agent and one of the most essential elements required for detox. If you consume soft drinks and other refined sweets during a detox programme, not only will they continuously acidify your blood and tissues when you're supposed to be alkalizing them, they'll also drain away all your vital calcium reserves, and force your body to leach additional calcium from your bones and teeth to combat the constant influx of acids. This defensive response to excess acidosisis in the bloodstream has become one of the main causes of osteoporosis, particularly in America, where people consume an astounding average of 53 teaspoons of refined white sugar per day, much of it in the form of carbonated soft drinks.

It's not just the sugar in soft drinks that makes them so dangerously acidifying to the blood and other bodily fluids. The carbonation in soft drinks is produced by forcing carbon dioxide gas into the sweet liquid and sealing it under pressure, so that when the can or bottle is opened, the gas is released as fizzy bubbles. As we already know, carbon dioxide is a waste product of human metabolism and a primary contributing factor to blood acidosis. To make matters even worse, the active ingredient in most of these fizzy sweet soft drinks is phosphoric acid, which has an extremely acid pH value of 2.8. Since human blood must maintain a slightly alkaline pH of 7.35 at all times, and even small flucuations can cause severe reactions, dropping an 'acid bomb' of sugar plus carbon dioxide plus phosphoric acid into your stomach causes a constant, rapid drain on your body's calcium resources. If you drink this stuff while trying to detox, its strong acid-forming properties will prevent your blood and tissues from ever reaching the degree of alkalinity required for the body's detox and healing mechanisms to switch on and function. Instead, your blood and tissues will remain in a constant state of acidosis, and rather than cleansing and repairing itself, your

body will be forced to fight a running biochemical battle just to
keep your blood pH from dropping to critically dangerous levels.

Alkaline à la carte

The basic purpose of a detox diet is to provide a highly alkalizing, totally non-acidifying source of nutrition that supports
the detox process whilst simultaneously producing as little
waste as possible in the body and requiring the least amount
of energy to digest. Everything consumed during detox should
specifically assist in alkalizing the body, purifying the bloodstream and detoxifying the tissues, while also helping to eliminate acid wastes and toxic residues through the excretory organs.
All of the manifold symptoms of blood and tissue toxicity, such
as chronic headaches and body pain, joint and tissue inflammation, bloating and swelling, indigestion and constipation, liver
congestion and nervous tension, respond quickly to a well
planned detox diet, which not only provides symptomatic relief
but also helps eliminate the root cause of all these conditions –
toxaemia.

The twin pillars of the detox diet are fresh fruit and fresh
vegetables. These must not only be fresh, they must also be
organically grown, non-genetically modified varieties, free of
chemical pesticides and irradiation. Any fruit or vegetable that
has been genetically modified, irradiated or grown with chemical pesticides and fertilizers is useless for detox purposes,
neither is it fit for daily human consumption. Fresh organic
produce, on the other hand, is a pure and potent source of alkalizing elements and antioxidant factors, as well as essential nutrients, to assist the detox and healing process. Fruits have
primarily cleansing and purging properties, while vegetables are
mainly curative and regenerative. Both are highly alkalizing,
produce very little waste, and don't require much energy or
many enzymes to digest. Together, fruit and vegetables provide

the full spectrum of nutritional and therapeutic elements required to detoxify and repair the body.

Fresh fruits are such a pure and simple form of food that most of them require no digestion whatsoever in the stomach. Instead, they move quickly into the duodenum, where they dissolve and release their nutrients for quick assimilation into the bloodstream within half an hour of ingestion. However, if there is any other food digesting in the stomach when fresh fruit is eaten, the fruit must back up and wait until the other food has been processed, before it can move on through to the duodenum. During this delay, the ever-present bacteria in the stomach feast on the fruit, metabolizing its nutrients and causing the fruit and everything else in the stomach to ferment rather than digest, producing toxic acid wastes and intestinal gas and upsetting the entire digestive tract. Fruit that would normally alkalize, nourish and cleanse the body thus becomes a source of acidosis, toxicity and indigestion instead. Therefore, the basic rule regarding fruit is, 'Eat it alone or leave it alone'. Some vegetables, especially when eaten raw, can take up to three hours to digest due to their high cellulose content, so fruit and vegetables should therefore always be consumed separately. In a detox diet, for example, vegetables may be included with the main meals at breakfast, lunch and dinner, and fruit eaten as snacks in between.

First, let's take a look at the vegetable section of the detox menu. The best choices in vegetables are those that actively cleanse and heal the body, alkalize the blood and tissues, and deliver optimum nutrition at minimum digestive cost. Such vegetables include sweet potatos, yams, squash, pumpkin, carrot, beetroot, cabbage, celery, parsley and all dark leafy greens. These items are rich not only in organic carotenes, which rank among the most powerful dietary healing factors, but also enzymes, minerals and various trace elements that are specifically beneficial in supporting the excretory functions of the liver, lungs, kidneys and bowels. Garlic, ginger and onion also have potent cleansing and curative

which helps support the excretory functions of the bowels and kidneys during detox.

Stir-frying This is definitely the best way to cook fresh vegetables as it preserves their fresh flavours and crisp textures, as well their nutritional value. The high heat softens the cell walls of the cellulose and cooks the vegetables just enough to make them easy to digest, while the short cooking time prevents their crispy textures from wilting and their bright colours from fading. When stir-frying vegetables, chopped ginger and garlic may be added to the pan together with the vegetables, but the salt should be added only at the very end of the cooking process. Root vegetables such as yams and beetroots are not really suitable for stir-frying, but squash, pumpkin and celery, as well as green leafy vegetables all lend themselves very well to stir-fry cooking. It's best to use only olive oil for stir-frying, because it provides the most beneficial forms of essential fatty acids and does not produce an abundance of free radicals at high cooking temperatures, as most other oils do. Good choices for stir-fried vegetables in the detox diet include spinach, kale, mustard greens, cabbage, bok choi, bamboo shoots and watercress. Watercress supplies abundant amounts of organic sulphur, calcium and magnesium and has particularly potent blood purifying properties. If your kidneys and bladder are ailing and need a cleansing alkaline flush-out, try stir-frying some tender fresh asparagus with ginger, garlic and sea salt. Asparagus is one of the most powerful natural alkalizers in the vegetable kingdom, and it flushes so much acid waste from the blood and kidneys so fast, that you can smell the ammonia in your urine within half an hour of eating it. If you prefer, asparagus may also be steamed for two or three minutes, rather than stir-fried.

Raw vegetable juice

To extract juice from fresh raw vegetables you need a proper vegetable extractor, which presses the juice from the vegetable cells under high pressure, extracting the essential fluid content and discarding the fibrous pulp. The great advantage of raw juice is that it retains all the potent active enzymes from the vegetables, which are destroyed by heat in the cooking process. Raw juice also preserves all of the vitamins and other essential nutrients in vegetables and delivers them into the stomach in ready-to-assimilate fluid form that requires no digestion. A glass of raw vegetable juice is the perfect complementary beverage for a detox meal of cooked vegetables: the juice provides the active enzymes and vitamins missing from the cooked vegetables, and the cooked vegetables provide the fibre removed from the juice.

Vegetable juices may be taken individually or blended in various combinations to provide specific therapeutic benefits to particular organs, glands and other tissues, by virtue of their natural pharmacodynamic affinity for specific parts of the body. There are now many good books available on raw juice therapy, and many health spas these days feature special 'juice bars' where guests can enjoy their 'Happy Hour' over a carrot and beetroot cocktail rather than a beer or whisky. A few tried-and-tested vegetable juices for detox are as follows:

Carrot This is perhaps the single most valuable vegetable juice for detox purposes. It cleanses the liver of stale bile and the stores of coagulated toxic residues that accumulate in the liver year after year as a result of eating chemically contaminated foods and wrong food combinations. Carrot juice provides abundant supplies of organic sulphur and chlorine for tissue cleansing purposes, calcium and magnesium to support the detox process, and natural carotenes, which provide strong antioxidant activity. Carrot is also the best base juice for blending special combinations with other juices.

Beetroot Beetroot juice is a potent cleanser of the liver and lower bowel. It also nourishes red blood cells, increases their capacity to carry oxygen and helps regulate menstrual cycles in women. Beetroot juice is quite strong and therefore only 50–100 ml, combined with 175–250 ml of carrot and/or other juices, should be taken per serving, and no more than 250 ml should be used per day.

Celery Celery juice is an excellent source of organic sodium chloride, which has strong cleansing and alkalizing properties and helps cool down the whole system. It's also a rich source of magnesium, which is required to produce alkaline enzymes for detox purposes. Celery juice is an effective remedy for disorders of the nervous system, including insomnia and nervous tension. Celery's nervine properties help keep body and mind relaxed and at ease during detox. A glass of fresh celery juice in the morning is a very good way to soothe a hangover after a long night of drinking, something that hopefully won't happen during a detox programme, but may come in handy at other times.

Parsley Parsley, like asparagus, is a powerful alkalizer with strong affinity for the kidneys and bladder. In addition to its potent kidney and bladder cleansing properties, parsley juice soothes and reduces inflammation in the urogenital canal and detoxifies the liver. It's a rich source of organic calcium and magnesium and helps purify the blood. In combination with carrot juice, parsley nourishes the eyes and improves vision. Parsley juice is strong medicine and should be taken only in combination with other juices, such as carrot. Don't use more than 75 ml a day.

Wheat grass juice If you have access to freshly extracted wheat grass juice, or if you're equipped to prepare it at home, it's highly recommended to include 50–75 ml a day in your detox diet, combined with carrot and other juices. Wheat grass juice is the ideal detox food: it provides fresh organic chlorophyll to purify the bloodstream and build strong blood, it alkalizes the blood and tissues, it contains the full range of essential amino acids, minerals and vitamins required for cellular regeneration, and it's brimming with active enzymes.

Breuss vegetable juice This is the juice recipe used in the cancer treatment developed by Rudolf Breuss, an Austrian health professional whose programme has helped more than 40,000 people cure themselves of cancer. It's also an excellent therapeutic blend for general detox purposes. To make enough juice for one day, put the following vegetables through a good juice extractor, then strain it through a fine sieve or muslin cloth to remove all sediment: 300 g beetroot, 100 g carrot, 100 g celeriac, 70 g potato, 30 g Chinese radish. You may drink a glass of this juice as part of a detox meal, or sip it slowly, 25 ml at a time, throughout the day as part of your detox diet. Breuss Vegetable Juice is also produced in bottled form by the Biotta company of Switzerland. Made only from organic, chemical-free vegetables and cold-pressed to preserve all the vital nutrients, enzymes and other healing factors, this is a pure, living vegetable juice that retains the therapeutic benefits and nutritional value of fresh raw juice. It's a very convenient way to take your vegetables during detox. In fact, two glasses per day of Breuss Vegetable Juice, either homemade or bottled from Biotta, is sufficient to provide all the nutritional support and alkalizing factors required during a detox programme.

Fresh fruits are the other mainstay of the detox diet, but not all fruits are suitable for detox purposes. The best choices for internal cleansing are citrus fruits and semi-sweet fruits from temperate climates such as apples, pears, watermelons, black cherries and black grapes. Tropical fruits such as mango, pineapple, banana and lychee have a very high content of fruit sugars and tend to overheat the system; the only exception is papaya, which facilitates detox and is particularly cleansing to the digestive tract owing to its rich content of active protease (protein-digesting) enzymes, which dissolve partially digested proteins and mucoid matter in the intestines. All fruits included in the detox diet should be organically grown and totally free of pesticides and other chemical sprays, and only fresh fruit should be eaten, not dried. As a result of the dehydration process, dried fruit contains much denser concentrations of fruit sugars and far fewer enzymes than fresh fruit, so the body has to expend its own energy and enzymes to process it. Fresh fruits, which are over 95 per cent water and contain their own active enzymes, virtually digest themselves.

There are three ways to eat fruit for detox purposes. One way is to extract the juice and strain out most of the pulp. This renders a very pure, highly alkalizing nectar that is easy to absorb and reaches the bloodstream quickly. A second way is to use a blender to make a 'fruit smoothie', but without adding any milk, yoghurt, soya milk, honey or any other ingredients – only fresh fruit and pure water. This produces a drink in which the juice is blended together with the puréed pulp, which provides an excellent source of hydrated fibre for the digestive tract. Thirdly, you may simply eat the fruit whole, with or without the peel. The peel of fruits such as apples, pears and grapes contain many valuable nutrients and healing factors, but they must be very well chewed in the mouth before swallowing in order to extract those nutrients, and the fruit must be certified organic to avoid poisoning yourself with the chemical sprays used on most commercial crops.

Many people are confused regarding the role of citrus fruits in maintaining a proper pH balance in the stomach and bloodstream. Citrus fruit juices are very cleansing to the stomach and digestive tract and help dissolve impacted mucus and putrefactive wastes, but if you measure the pH value of any citrus juice with litmus paper, you'll find that it falls decisively into the acid range. However, the pH value of a food outside the stomach does not determine whether it has acid-forming or alkaline-forming effects within the stomach; what counts is how a particular food *reacts* with the digestive juices and other foods in the stomach after it's eaten, and whether it acidifies or alkalizes the bloodstream after it's digested. In the case of citrus fruits, if they are eaten on an empty stomach and allowed to pass unobstructed into the duodenum, they become highly alkalizing and very beneficial for internal cleansing and detox. However, if you drink a glass of orange or grapefruit juice with a meal of toast, eggs, pancakes and/or cereal – as millions of people do every day when eating a modern Western-style breakfast – the citrus juice, unable to pass into the duodenum, sits on top of the other food and quickly ferments, preventing the proper digestion of everything else in the stomach and turning it all into a frothing fermentive stew that causes gas, forms acid wastes and increases tissue toxicity. Therefore, in order to gain maximum benefit from their cleansing and alkalizing properties, and to avoid their acid-forming reactions with other foods, citrus fruits should always be eaten separately from any other foods, including all other types of fruit.

As with all items in the detox diet, the fewer your choices in fruit, and the more simply you combine them, the better they will work to purify your blood, detoxify your tissues and cleanse your digestive tract. Here are a few suggestions:

Apples Apples aid digestion and cleanse the intestinal tract, and may be eaten either whole or juiced. Apple cores are very rich in pectin, which acts as a potent intestinal detoxificant, and raw apple juice usually reduces the fever and tissue inflammation that sometimes occur during detox as it helps dislodge heavy toxins and release them into the bloodstream for excretion. Another raw apple product that may be used for detox purposes is organic apple cider vinegar. Unlike all other vinegars, which contain acetic acid and are therefore acid-forming, apple cider vinegar contains malic acid, which is alkalizing to the body. Two tablespoons of apple cider vinegar with one teaspoon of raw honey stirred into a glass of warm water may be taken once or twice a day, before meals, to cleanse the stomach and balance pH throughout the digestive system. This is particularly beneficial for those who suffer from gastritis.

Pears Pears are loaded with alkalizing elements and have a natural affinity for the kidneys, where they provide a gentle diuretic effect, cleanse them, and dissolve crystalized acid residues before they can form kidney stones.

Grapes The best type of grapes for detox purposes are black grapes. The juice of raw black grapes is known among vegans as 'vegetarian milk' because of its capacity to sustain nursing infants deprived of mother's milk, without using dairy milk. Black grapes are particularly effective for treating constipation and gastritis, detoxifying the liver and kidneys, and purifying the blood. In Russia, there are entire clinics devoted exclusively to what they call 'The Grape Cure', where patients are fed nothing but raw black grapes for up to a month or more. This regimen has been effectively used to cure various forms of cancer, heart disease, hepatitis, nervous system disorders and many other serious conditions that conventional medicine often views as 'incurable'. Glucose, which is also known as 'blood sugar' and is the main form of sugar found in grapes, is the body's primary metabolic fuel and is especially important for brain functions. Since grapes directly provide the bloodstream with the precise form of fuel required by the cells, they help curb the craving for rich foods that often manifests when you're trying to restrict your diet to just a few simple items. The skins and seeds of grapes are also rich in nutrients and cleansing factors, but they must be chewed very well in order to release these elements for assimilation. If you don't have the patience to chew the skins and seeds of whole grapes, you may purée them whole in a blender, which does the chewing job for you. Like all fruit, grapes should be eaten at least one or two hours apart from vegetables and other foods. If you choose to eat nothing else but grapes for your detox diet, you may eat as many of them as you wish from morning till night.

Citrus Oranges, grapefruits and lemons are wonderful alkalizers and cleansers when consumed alone, either whole or juiced. They help dissolve mucus and phlegm throughout the system, alkalize the blood and bodily fluids, and decongest the liver. Fresh grapefruit is extraordinarily rich in salicylic acid, which dissolves crystallized calcium deposits in the joints, thereby relieving arthritis. In conjunction with long-term reforms in daily diet after a few detox programs, arthritis can be gradually and permanently cured with grapefruit therapy. Citrus juice also has strong antiseptic and antifungal properties, which can be important during detox. Never add sugar or any other sweetener to fresh citrus juice because any additive will cause it to ferment in the stomach and become highly acid-forming, rather than alkalizing. Always consume citrus fruits and juices separately from other foods, on an empty stomach.

Watermelon Watermelon is an excellent internal organ cleanser, especially for the kidneys and bladder. When eaten whole, it should be cut up into bite-sized chunks and chewed slowly, bite by bite, throughout the day. Alternatively, it may be puréed in a blender, including the white rind, which contains potent kidney cleansing factors. Watermelon is one of the most alkalizing of fruits and, owing to its natural affinity for the kidneys, it helps dissolve and prevent the formation of kidney stones.

Papaya Papaya's abundant supply of protease enzymes makes it particularly effective as a digestive aid and detoxifying agent for bowels that are clogged with putrefactive protein wastes from excessive consumption of meat, eggs and dairy products. Papaya also stimulates secretions of digestive juices in the stomach and duodenum, and when there's nothing else in the stomach, these digestive enzymes travel down to dissolve mucus and break down putrid waste matter in the intestines.

Grains and nuts

Almost all major grain foods are acid-forming and require a lot of energy and enzymes to digest, so they should either be eliminated entirely, or else strictly limited in the detox diet. The only major grain food that is alkaline-forming is millet, so this is the best choice when grains are included in the detox diet. If millet is unavailable, the next best options, in order of preference, are spelt, barley, rye, buckwheat or brown rice. All wheat products should be eliminated completely: not only is wheat one of the most acid-forming grains, it also causes allergic reactions in many people, which can become particularly severe during detox.

Only whole, organically grown grains should be included in the detox diet, and absolutely no flour products, such as bread, pasta and pastry. The grain should be washed well and pre-soaked in pure water for at least 6 hours, or overnight, then boiled for a few hours with plenty of water and a teaspoon of sea salt, until it forms a thin gruel, or porridge. In Chinese, this sort of watery boiled grain is called *hsi-fan*, literally 'diluted rice', or 'congee'. During cooking, if the gruel becomes too thick, stir in another cup or so of water. Millet makes an excellent gruel, and so do barley and brown rice. An even better choice is a tasty medicinal grain called Job's tears (*Coix lacryma-jobi*), or *yi-yi-ren* in Chinese, which has diuretic properties, decongests the lungs, eliminates phlegm and removes excess dampness from the joints and tissues. A simple recipe for Job's tears and brown rice porridge is given in the Recipes and Formulas section in Appendix 1 on page 326.

Thin gruel made from whole grain is relatively easy to digest and provides a variety of essential nutrients, including a variety of B vitamins, minerals and amino acids. Gruel also adds fibrous bulk to the diet to facilitate bowel movements, and provides carbohydrates for metabolic energy. As noted above, it's generally best to abstain from grain during detox and save the digestive energy and enzymes for internal cleansing purposes instead. In some cases, however, such as liver and nerve detox, it's helpful to include a limited amount of whole grains gruel as a source of B vitamins, amino acids, and other factors that are of specific benefit to liver and nerve tissue.

Note that all grains become alkaline-forming when sprouted. Sprouting transforms them into complete living foods bursting with essential nutrients, active enzymes and energy. Therefore, freshly sprouted grains may always be included with the main meals in a detox diet.

Raw nuts and seeds are an excellent source of vegetable protein, essential fatty acids, vitamins and minerals, but in order to digest them and extract their nutritional benefits, raw nuts and seeds must be pre-soaked overnight in pure water before you eat them. All nuts and seeds have a special 'anti-digestive' factor built into them, specifically designed by nature to prevent them from rotting (i.e. digesting themselves). That's why they may be kept unrefrigerated for a long time without decaying. However, if you eat them like that, this natural preservative factor also prevents your stomach from properly digesting them, and consequently they ferment instead, producing gas and acid wastes. When raw nuts and seeds are pre-soaked overnight, the water eliminates the anti-digestive factor and signals the nut or seed to 'wake up', just as it would if the nut or seed were planted in the ground and watered. While soaking in water overnight, nuts and seeds come to life and release their rich reserves of nutrients and other health factors. When you eat them like this, they become very easy to digest, and all of their abundant nutritional potential becomes available for assimilation.

Like grains, however, most nuts and seeds are acid-forming in the body and should therefore not be eaten during detox. Fortunately, the only exception is the most beneficial nut of all, the almighty almond, which is not only alkalizing to the human system, but also ranks as one of the very best foods in nature for human health and longevity. Almonds are one of the purest, most potent sources of the essential amino acids and fatty acids that form the 'bricks and mortar' of cell and tissue construction;

they also provide abundant amounts of other vital nutrient co-factors, particularly calcium and magnesium – the 'dynamic duo' of mineral elements for detox. Heaven only knows what other unknown healing factors lie hidden in almonds, waiting to be discovered; the famous clairvoyant healer Edgar Cayce, who successfully diagnosed and cured thousands of severely sick people, often said that anyone who eats a few raw almonds every day will never develop cancer.

To prepare almonds for eating, use only raw, preferably organically grown whole almonds that have been shelled but not blanched. Place them in a bowl, cover with pure water, and set aside to soak overnight. Next morning, drain off the water, and the almonds are ready to eat. It's a good idea to peel off the brown skins, which are very easy to remove after the nuts have been soaked, because any contaminants to which the nuts have been exposed will have been trapped in the skin. Soaked almonds remain fresh and ready to eat all day; any left-overs should be kept in the refrigerator and may still be eaten the next day. Soaked almonds are so satisfying to the appetite, so easy to digest and so rich in nutritional value that including them as a staple in the detox diet makes it relatively easy to abstain from the heavy, acid-forming foods, such as meat and dairy products, bread and pasta, that most people normally eat as staples in their daily diet. By depending on almonds during detox, you may even grow so fond of their fine flavour and crunchy texture that you'll start substituting almonds for some of the heavier, acid-forming foods permanently.

Detox beverages

What you drink is as much a part of your diet as what you eat, and in a detox diet, water and other liquid nourishment are particularly important. In order to continuously flush toxins out the kidneys and replenish all bodily fluids with pure water, you must drink *at least* 6–8 glasses (1.5–2 litres) of pure, preferably alkaline and ionized, water each and every day throughout the duration of a detox programme. This is absolutely essential for success. A glass of fruit or vegetable juice, or a cup of herbal tea, does not count as a glass of water just because it's fluid and contains water. Juices and teas function in an entirely different way in the human body to pure water, and only water that is consumed 'straight' can purify the blood, detoxify the tissues, rehydrate the cells and replenish the bodily fluids. Water should be consumed separately from food, not with meals, and the first two glasses should be taken immediately upon arising in the morning, before eating anything, to flush mucus and food residues from the stomach and digestive tract. Drink another glass or two between breakfast and lunch, and again between lunch and dinner, and the last one between dinner and bedtime.

Another important beverage during detox is herbal tea. Herbal teas are very useful supports for various aspects of the detoxi-fication and purification process, enhancing the functions of the organs and glands involved and relieving the symptomatic discomforts of detox. Almost all herbal teas are alkalizing and have therapeutic benefits for detox, so may be sipped freely throughout the day. Depending on which organs and tissues require the most attention during a detox programme, you may select specific herbal teas that have what TCM refers to as 'natural affinity' (*gui jing*) for those particular organs and tissues, such as using dandelion and milk thistle to detoxify the liver, horsetail and nettle to clean the kidneys, or valerian and passion flower to soothe the nerves, and so forth. A variety of herbal teas and other herbal formulas that may be used as supplements to help detoxify specific organs and tissues and relieve the discomforts of detox are presented in Chapter 8, Herbal Detox, and you may include a selection of these in any detox programme, according to your personal requirements.

One herbal tea that is generally beneficial for all detox and internal cleansing purposes and may therefore be included in all detox programmes is sage tea, which plays a central role in the Breuss cancer cure (see p.180), An old Roman proverb asks, 'Why die, when there is sage in the garden?' Sage has been used since ancient times for its potent cleansing and healing properties, and as an effective preventive medicine against disease and degeneration. It contains factors that nourish all of the glands as well as the spinal cord, thereby helping the body to produce the hormones and neurochemicals involved in cleansing, healing and regenerating the whole system. A large vacuum flask full of hot sage tea may be prepared first thing each morning and taken as desired throughout the day and evening. The recipe for this excellent herbal detox tea is given in Recipes and Formulas on page 327.

Detox supplements

To fortify the detox diet with extra cleansing and healing power, various nutritional supplements may be included to selectively assist different dimensions of the detox process, and to target specific organs and tissues for extra attention. Only supplements made from natural food concentrates and pure plant or mineral extracts should be included in the detox diet, and anything synthesized from chemicals or other artificial ingredients should be strictly avoided.

Supplements serve three basic purposes in the detox diet: they help alkalize the blood and tissues, thereby maintaining the internal 'climate' of alkalinity required for cleansing and healing responses to function properly; they provide additional supplies of antioxidants, chlorophyll, carotenes and other essential detoxifying elements; and they supply extra reserves of vital detox nutrients, especially the all-important vitamin and mineral factors that are so centrally involved in the myriad metabolic enzyme reactions that occur during detox. A few of the most useful detox supplements are briefly introduced below:

Minerals

It's a good idea to include some form of full-spectrum, easily assimilated mineral supplement in all detox programmes, and the best choice for this purpose is seawater, which may be taken straight from clean ocean waters or as a concentrated fluid extract of pure marine minerals. Another good source is home-made bittern of Celtic sea salt, or ⅓ teaspoon of Celtic sea salt dissolved in a glass of pure water. Seawater and sea salt contain the full range of minerals and trace elements required by the body, and in precisely the proper proportions. In fact, the mineral composition and pH value of human blood and natural seawater are virtually identical.

In addition to full-spectrum mineral supplementation, the body also requires extra amounts of calcium and magnesium during detox. Calcium is the body's primary alkalizing agent, and it's also needed for balanced functioning of all the major organ systems, including the nervous system. It's involved in every major metabolic reaction and is essential for new cell growth and tissue regeneration. An excellent source of this macro-mineral is coral calcium, which is exceptionally alkalizing and relatively easy to assimilate. Simply dissolve the powder in pure water and take it two or three times daily, with or without food.

Magnesium is a key component in a wide range of alkaline enzymes that the body must produce to conduct the detox process, and it's also a vital factor for balancing heart and nervous system functions. Calcium and magnesium work together as the 'dynamic duo' of detox, and it's important to obtain sufficient quantities of both in order for either one to be completely effective. The easiest form of magnesium to assimilate is magnesium chloride, as found in the sea, and an excellent source of this is the magnesium-rich bittern extracted from Celtic sea salt, which you can easily prepare at home as described in Chapter 2 on page 50. Alternatively, you may use concentrated marine mineral extracts derived from pure seawater, available at many health shops or by mail order.

Green food

Green food refers to any purified food concentrate made from the freshly extracted juice of young cereal grasses, such as wheat, rye and barley, or extracted from water plants and green algae that grow on the surface of large, unpolluted lakes. They are called 'green' due to their high concentration of pure organic chlorophyll, which is one of nature's most potent blood purifiers and tissue cleansers and a 'must' for any detox programme. It's an interesting and significant fact of nature that, with the sole exception of a single molecule, the chlorophyll in plants and the haemoglobin in human blood have precisely the same biochemical composition. The only difference is that where haemoglobin has a molecule of iron, chlorophyll has a molecule of magnesium.

Haemoglobin is the factor in blood that's responsible for carrying oxygen, and without sufficient haemoglobin, the blood's capacity to carry oxygen diminishes rapidly, reducing its power to detoxify and nourish the tissues. Chlorophyll builds strong haemoglobin and swiftly purifies the bloodstream, thereby supporting the entire detox process by enhancing the blood's capacity to hold oxygen and deliver it to the tissues. As Dr Bernard Jensen, one of the leading authorities on detox therapy, states, 'Chlorophyll can speed up the rate of cleansing the bowel, bloodstream, and liver.' Since cleansing the bowel, bloodstream and liver represents about 75 per cent of the work in detox, chlorophyll is the sovereign element for getting the detox job done swiftly and effectively.

Green food also contains the full range of essential amino acids required for reproducing cells and repairing tissues, as well all the essential vitamins, minerals and enzymes that the body needs to cleanse and heal itself. Green food supplies all of these elements in their purest, most bio-available forms. As a nutritionally complete food as well as a rich source of blood and tissue cleansing factors, green food may be used as the sole form of nutrition during a detox programme, without the need for any other type of food. Since green foods are pure, highly concentrated extracts of living plants, they're loaded with active enzymes and therefore digest themselves without requiring any additional energy or enzymes from your body, and their nutrients are rapidly released for immediate assimilation into the bloodstream and swift delivery to the cells and tissues. This means they produce virtually no acid wastes in the body – an obvious advantage during detox – while still delivering the full range of essential nutrients in the purest, most readily utilized form possible in any food.

The juice of young cereal grasses, such as wheat and barley, is one of the most widely used green foods for detox purposes, and it may be taken either freshly extracted (which requires a special machine) or in the form of the dried powder pressed into tablets. One of the best wheat grass supplements on the market today is called Green Life, made in America by the V.E. Irons Co. as part of their excellent line of Vit-ra-tox internal cleansing products. Green Life is made from the dried, cold-extracted juices of organically grown cereal grasses, including wheat, barley, oats and rye, and is available either as loose powder or pressed tablets. It also contains powdered extract of whole beetroot juice to detoxify the liver and bowels, sea kelp to rebuild the blood and papaya enzymes to dissolve putrefactive proteins and impacted dried mucoid matter in the intestinal tract. This product contains all the elements required by the body to detoxify and purify itself, including 50,000 IU of natural beta-carotene per 100 g portion, almost double the amount found in fresh carrots. In addition, it contains about 25 per cent pure vegetable protein, including a properly balanced blend of 20 natural amino acids, to help build new cells and repair damaged tissues.

Another excellent green food supplement is Barley Green, produced by AIM International in the USA. This comes in a light green powder that may be stirred into juice or water, or swallowed dry by the spoonful and washed down with juice or water. Extracted from pure barley grass, it's densely packed with chlorophyll, nutrients and active enzymes in highly concentrated form.

Spirulina, blue-green algae and chlorella are examples of green foods made from the simple, single-celled aquatic plants that grow on the surfaces of large unpolluted lakes located in pristine mountains and forest regions. These organisms are among the oldest forms of life on earth, having first appeared about two billion years ago, when plant life still ruled the planet. Their nutritional profile includes an amazing 58 g of pure vegetable protein and a whopping 2.1 g of pure organic chlorophyll per 100 serving. Like the green foods derived from cereal grasses, spirulina and other micro-algae also provide all the essential B vitamins required for detox and healing, including the highest known vegetable source of vitamin B_{12}, which is very difficult to obtain from any other non-animal food source. B vitamins are particularly important for repairing and rebalancing the liver, brain and nervous system, and since the normal dietary sources of these vitamins are grains and animal products, which are highly acid-forming and should be avoided during detox, green foods provide a convenient alternative source of these essential nutritional factors in a pure, potent form that alkalizes rather than acidifies the body.

Treacle
Natural unsulphured treacle is one of the richest and most easily assimilated sources of essential minerals in balanced organic form. The roots of sugar cane can grow as deep as 5–6 metres into the ground, allowing them to tap into the abundant reserves of minerals that lie beneath the depleted topsoil and remain out

of reach of other crops. Since mineralization of blood and tissues is one of the primary strategies in all detox programmes, treacle is a convenient and effective supplement for this purpose, especially for people with long-term mineral deficiency. Treacle is one of the best natural sources of organic iron as well as copper, which is an essential co-factor for the utilization of iron in the body. This makes it an excellent supplement for building strong blood, and a good tonic for those suffering from anaemia. In addition, treacle provides lots of calcium and magnesium, both of which the body needs extra supplies of during detox.

Alkaline vitamin C

Alkaline vitamin C, or 'C-salts', is a non-acidic form of vitamin C bound to various alkaline mineral salts. This allows it to be used in large dosages without the acidifying effects produced by the more common, less expensive acetic acid form of vitamin C. Vitamin C is both a potent antioxidant and an important nutrient that plays an indispensable metabolic role in the detox process. It's thus a good idea to include a supplemental source of alkaline vitamin C in all detox programmes. Calcium ascorbate and sodium ascorbate are the two most widely used C-salts, and both are available in tablet or pure powdered form; the latter may be stirred into water or juice throughout the day. A suitable dosage for most detox purposes is 3–5g per day, although it may also be taken in much larger amounts for additional antioxidant activity.

Liquid bentonite

Also known as 'clay water', bentonite is a super-fine, colloidal form of volcanic ash consisting of micro-molecules that are 500 times smaller than water molecules, and each one carries a strong negative charge. These molecules saturate the blood and bodily fluids, penetrating places where even water cannot go, and they act like millions of micro-magnets to attract and neutralize positively charged toxic molecules lodged deeply in tissues and fluids throughout the body. The neutralized toxins are then carried away in the bloodstream for excretion. A single molecule of bentonite can adsorb 200 times its own weight in toxic wastes, and its cleansing action is entirely mechanical, producing no chemical reactions whatsoever in the body. One of the best grades of liquid bentonite on the market is the Vitra-tox label, which may be ordered by mail from the address provided in the Suppliers section in Appendix 2. One tablespoon of bentonite stirred into a glass of water and taken 2–3 times per day, separately from food, is an adequate dosage for most detox programmes, although double this amount may be taken in extreme cases of blood and tissue toxicity. If you're also using psyllium, take the bentonite as a 'chaser' immediately after the psyllium.

Psyllium seed
The ground seed and husk of psyllium (*Plantago ovato blond*), known in India as 'flea seed', is by far the most effective natural fibre bulking supplement for clearing clogged bowels of impacted faeces, dry mucoid plaque and putrefactive food residues. There is no better remedy for chronic constipation and sluggish bowels than ground psyllium, which, like liquid bentonite, functions entirely on a mechanical basis, without causing any chemical reactions whatsoever. One teaspoon of ground psyllium shaken well with about 300 ml of water and drunk down quickly on an empty stomach forms a dense, mucilagenous bolus that sweeps like a broom throughout the entire digestive tract, loosening and eliminating pockets of impacted putrefactive waste and mucoid sludge from the deep folds of the colon. Psyllium facilitates regular bowel movements, dredges the colon of dangerous toxic residues that have festered there for years, and accelerates the entire detox process. One or two doses per day on an empty stomach is sufficient when using

psyllium as a supplement in the detox diet, but when fasting, four doses per day should be taken in order to provide a constant cleansing action within the bowels. Always remember to drink an extra glass of water immediately after taking a dose of psyllium, and if you're also using bentonite, add it to the second glass of water. The ground psyllium seed powder produced by Vit-ra-tox as part of its line of detox supplements is called Intestinal Cleanser and is one of the best on the market today. Another excellent variety of this important detox supplement is Herbal Fibre Blend, produced under the AIM label. This is a balanced blend of 18 cleansing herbs combined in a base of ground psyllium. The herbs eliminate intestinal parasites, stimulate excretory functions, detoxify the internal organs and rebalance the entire digestive system.

Cayenne

Cayenne is one of the most effective healing herbs on earth, and it has strong cleansing properties that greatly assist the detox process. Cayenne gives a big boost to blood circulation and balances heart functions, thereby ensuring sufficient supplies of oxygen and nutrients to all tissues. In addition, cayenne stimulates the entire endocrine system, strengthens immune response, clears liver congestion, activates peristalsis and lower bowel functions, and energizes the whole digestive system. Believe it or not, cayenne is also one of the best remedies for stomach ulcers: it cleanses and disinfects the ulcers and promotes their rapid healing. On top of all that, cayenne is highly alkalizing, which makes it a perfect detox supplement, especially for those with circulatory and heart problems, stomach ulcers and/or stagnant digestive systems. One or two capsules taken once or twice a day with a glass of warm water is an effective therapeutic dosage for detox purposes. Cayenne is most effective taken on an empty stomach, but it may also be taken with meals to buffer the heat it produces in the stomach. You can quickly quell the heat of cayenne taken between meals by eating an apple with it.

Lemon

Fresh lemon is the only food in the world that is anionic, which means it carries a negative molecular charge. This does not apply to other citrus fruits such as lime or grapefruit, only to fresh lemon, the juice of which must be consumed freshly extracted in order to retain its detoxifying anionic properties. The negative charge combined with its strong alkalizing effects makes fresh lemon juice one of the most powerful detoxifying supplements of all, and it may be used to assist any type of detox programme. It should always be taken on an empty stomach, mixed into a glass of pure water, without the addition of any sweeteners. Fresh lemon juice assists the production of bile in the liver, and without adequate bile production, it's impossible to properly digest food and assimilate nutrients. An excellent way to use fresh lemon juice as a detox supplement is to blend it with ground whole flaxseed, alkaline vitamin C powder and selected herbs to make a lemon flax shake. This may be taken twice daily, between meals, throughout the duration of a detox programme. The recipe is given in the Recipes and Formulas section on page 327.

Daily detox menus

The dietary guidelines given in this chapter, including the sample menus presented below, are specifically designed for detox purposes, not for daily life. Since one tries to remain calm and quiet during detox, resting in a state of uninterrupted relaxation and avoiding all stress and strain that might activate the 'fight or flight' response, while also refraining from strenuous muscular exertion that produces lactic acid in the tissues, the body requires far fewer calories during detox than it does in daily life. Moreover, detox requires a diet that produces minimal acid wastes and consumes minimal digestive energy, while delivering maximum nutrition and providing precisely the elements the body needs to detoxify and cleanse itself. Such a diet does not meet the requirements of daily life for an active person, because it does not provide sufficient calories to generate the energy required for an active lifestyle, nor does it contain the proper mixture of food elements the body needs for daily life. The detox diet outlined in this chapter should therefore only be used for the specific purpose of deliberately detoxifying the body, preferably in conjunction with other detox modalities introduced in this book, for periods of three days up to three weeks. After that, if you wish to reform your diet so that it protects your health and prolongs your life by producing minimum toxicity and providing maximum nutrition, you may adopt some of the dietary suggestions offered in the chapter on Retox Diet and Supplements in Part 2 of this book.

As a general guideline to assist the reader in composing his or her own daily menus for detox programmes of three days to three weeks duration, six sample detox menus are presented for reference below. These menus are geared to various different appetites, tastes and detox requirements, and each one focuses primary therapeutic attention on particular organs and tissues that need the most work. Feel free to mix and match the recommended foods and supplements in whatever way best suits your own personal tastes and individual therapeutic needs, as long as you do not include any items or combinations that are counterproductive to detox and healing.

Generally speaking, the more fluid and fewer solid, the more raw and fewer cooked, the more nutrient-dense and fewer calorie-rich items you include in your detox diet, the more detoxifying that diet becomes and the more effectively it heals your body. It's important to remember that in the detox diet, 'less is more': the less you eat, the more you detox. In fact, the best detox diet of all is fasting, as we shall see in the following chapter. Therefore, please do not feel obliged to follow strictly the suggestions below when designing your own personal detox programme. Instead, use them as general dietary guidelines to help you compose menus that satisfy your own therapeutic requirements without overly offending your basic tastes in food. Once you've decided on a particular detox menu, it's best not to stray too far from it for the duration of your programme. The simpler and more consistent you make it, the better it will work for you.

A few basic items should be included in all the detox menus suggested below. Most important of all is to drink at least 6–8 glasses (1.5–2 litres) of pure alkaline water each and every day, as follows: 2 glasses immediately upon arising in the morning; 1–2 glasses between breakfast and lunch; 2–3 glasses between lunch and dinner; and 1 glass between dinner and bedtime. Sage tea is recommended for general cleansing and healing purposes in all these detox menus, in addition to various other herbal teas for specific conditions. Some form of full-spectrum mineral supplement, such as marine minerals or Celtic sea salt, is recomended in all menus, as well as some type of 'green food', such as wheat or barley grass juice, spirulina or chlorella. Other supplements may be included to enhance various aspects of the detox process according to your own individual requirements.

Menu 1

Therapeutic focus General tissue detox

Breakfast: Steamed pumpkin with shredded ginger and Celtic sea salt
Veg. Juice: 250 ml fresh Breuss Vegetable Juice or bottled Biotta brand
8–12 pre-soaked raw almonds

Mid-morning snack:	Fresh apples and/or black grapes
Lunch:	Half a fresh avocado with chopped garlic, Celtic sea salt, and olive oil
	Veg. juice: 250 ml fresh Breuss blend or Biotta brand
Mid-afternoon snack:	Fresh papaya or watermelon juice
Dinner:	Spinach or watercress stir-fried with ginger and garlic
	Millet or Job's Tears and brown rice gruel
Evening snack:	Fresh apples and/or black grapes
Herb tea:	Sage tea
Supplements:	Green food, 3× a day with meals
	Marine minerals and coral calcium, 1–2× a day, with meals
	Psyllium seed, 1–2× a day, on an empty stomach

Remarks Avocado may be eaten as it is, rather than as juice, because the flesh does not contain tough cellulose; it is a rich source of essential fatty acids, vegetable protein and other nutrients, and provides abundant fuel for metabolic energy. If arthritis is a problem, use freshly squeezed grapefruit juice rather than other fruits for the three snacks; grapefruit is one of the best sources of organic salicylic acid, which dissolves inorganic calcium deposits from the joints.

Menu 2

Therapeutic focus Bowels and digestive tract

Breakfast:	Stewed vegetables: carrot, pumpkin, turnip, squash
	Clear vegetable broth with miso paste
	12–15 pre-soaked raw almonds
Mid-morning snack:	Fresh papaya, apples
Lunch:	12–15 pre-soaked raw almonds
	Veg. juice: 200 ml carrot, 100 ml beetroot
Afternoon snack:	Fresh papaya, apples
Dinner:	Steamed okra with chopped garlic, ginger, and Celtic sea salt
	Half a fresh avocado with garlic, Celtic sea salt, and olive oil
	Clear vegetable broth with miso paste
Evening snack:	Black grapes
Herb tea:	Sage tea
Supplements:	Psyllium seed, 2× a day, on an empty stomach
	Liquid bentonite, 2× a day, immediately after psyllium
	Cayenne, 1 cap. 2× a day, with lunch and dinner
	Green food, 3× a day, with meals
	Aloe vera juice, fresh or bottled, 1–2× a day

Remarks Cooked vegetables and whole raw fruits provide plenty of natural fibre to help dredge wastes from the bowels, and okra is particularly effective for cleansing the colon and facilitating bowel movements. Miso provides a rich source of active enzymes to assist in the digestion of putrefactive wastes lodged in the bowels. Psyllium supplies additional pure vegetable fibre to loosen and eliminate impacted mucoid wastes, while bentonite absorbs toxic particles released from the lining of the digestive tract by the psyllium. Cayenne cleanses and heals ulcers in the stomach and intestinal tract, and aloe vera juice is one of nature's most effective digestive tract cleansers, as well as an excellent remedy for constipation and colitis.

Menu 3

Therapeutic focus Heart and circulatory system

Breakfast:	Half a fresh avocado with olive oil
	Veg. juice: 200 ml carrot, 50 ml spinach, 50 ml celery, 8–12 pre-soaked raw almonds
Mid-morning snack:	Fresh orange juice
Lunch:	Spinach or watercress stir-fried with garlic
	Steamed pumpkin with ginger
Mid-afternoon snack:	Fresh orange juice or black grapes
Dinner:	Millet or barley or Job's Tears and brown rice gruel
	Stir-fried leafy greens with garlic
	Veg. juice: 300 ml carrot

Evening snack:	Apples and/or black grapes
Herb tea:	Sage tea; hawthorn berry tea
Supplements:	Marine minerals and coral calcium, 1× a day, before breakfast
	Cayenne, 1 cap. 2× a day, with lunch and dinner
	CoQ10, 60 mg daily, after breakfast
	Green food, 2× a day, with breakfast and dinner
	Hawthorn berry extract, 1–2× a day, in warm water, between meals

Remarks Garlic helps cleanse the blood vessels and remove plaque, while cayenne is the single most beneficial herb for regulating heart function, balancing pulse and stimulating blood circulation. Marine minerals provide the essential trace elements required by the heart and bloodstream to regulate blood pressure; green food purifies the bloodstream and increases the blood's capacity to carry oxygen; and raw almonds are a rich source of organic calcium and magnesium. Hawthorn berry fortifies the heart muscle and coronary vessels and helps stabilize heartbeat, and CoQ10 has been shown to help correct imbalances in heart function.

Menu 4

Therapeutic focus Brain and nervous system

| **Breakfast:** | 12–15 pre-soaked raw almonds |
| | Clear vegetable broth |

	Steamed pumpkin with ginger and Celtic sea salt
Mid-morning snack:	Black cherries and/or black grapes
Lunch:	Millet or barley or Job's Tears and brown rice gruel
	Spinach or watercress or kale stir-fried with garlic and Celtic sea salt
	Veg. juice: 200 ml carrot, 100 ml celery
Mid-afternoon snack:	Fresh apples and/or pears
	Black cherries and/or black grapes
Dinner:	Millet or barley or Job's Tears and brown rice gruel
	Stewed vegetables
	Veg. juice: 100 ml carrot, 50 ml celery
Evening snack:	Apples and/or pears
Herb tea:	Sage tea; camomile tea; passion flower and lemon balm tea
Supplements:	Nervine herbal formulas (see Chapter 8), 2× a day, between meals
	Coriander cilantro extract, 2–3× a day, between meals
	Gingko biloba, 2× a day, after breakfast and lunch
	Marine minerals, 2× a day, before breakfast and dinner

Remarks Concentrated extract of coriander is a potent detoxifier of brain cells and nerve tissue, and it is especially effective for removing heavy metal toxins. Gingko biloba provides powerful antioxidant activity in the brain and nerves and also increases micro-circulation in the brain. The body requires B vitmains to detoxify and repair nerve and brain tissue, and these are provided by the gruel, almonds and green food. Celery juice contains elements that calm the nervous system and relieve insomnia. Marine minerals and sea salt provide the full spectrum of essential minerals and trace elements which the brain and nervous system need to function properly, and the nervine herbal teas and extracts keep the nervous system relaxed, prevent anxiety from developing during the detox process, and promote sound sleep.

Menu 5

Therapeutic focus Kidneys and bladder

Breakfast:	Veg. juice: 200 ml carrot, 60 ml beetroot, 40 ml parsley, 8–12 pre-soaked raw almonds Clear vegetable broth with miso paste
Mid-morning snack:	Fresh watermelon, cut into small bite-sized pieces and eaten slowly
Lunch:	Veg. juice: 250 ml fresh Breuss vegetable juice or bottled Biotta brand Watercress stir-fried with garlic
Mid-afternoon snack:	Fresh watermelon, small pieces eaten slowly

Dinner:	Steamed or poached fresh asparagus with garlic and Celtic sea salt
	Millet gruel
	Veg. juice: 100 ml carrot, 30 ml beetroot, 20 ml parsley
Evening snack:	Black cherries or black grapes
Herb tea:	Sage tea; Breuss kidney tea
Supplements:	Green food, 2× a day, with breakfast and dinner
	Marine minerals or Celtic sea salt bittern, 2× a day, before breakfast and dinner

Remarks Asparagus has strong cleansing effects on the kidneys and bladder, flushing out acid wastes so fast that you can smell the ammonia in your urine shortly after eating it. Parsley purifies and protects kidney tissues, which is especially important when the kidneys are working overtime to excrete toxic wastes. It's important to drink plenty of water when cleansing the kidneys, and better to eat more fluid and fewer solid foods. Eating fresh watermelon slowly produces a steady stream of cleansing elements that flow through the kidneys and bladder, detoxifying and soothing inflammation in those tissues.

Menu 6

Therapeutic focus Liver and blood

| **Breakfast:** | Steamed pumpkin with ginger and Celtic sea salt |
| | Veg. juice: 200 ml carrot, 50 ml beetroot, 8–12 pre-soaked raw almonds |

Mid-morning snack:	Black grapes
Lunch:	Veg. juice: fresh tomato, 200 ml
	Job's Tears and brown rice gruel
	Steamed pumpkin (leftover from breakfast)
Mid-afternoon snack:	Black grapes
Dinner:	Spinach or watercress stir-fried with garlic and Celtic sea salt
	Veg. juice: 200 ml carrot, 50 ml beetroot
	Job's Tears and brown rice gruel
Evening snack:	Black grapes
Herb tea:	Sage tea; milk thistle and dandelion tea; liquorice root and chrysanthemum tea
Supplements:	Bentonite, 2× a day between meals
	Green food, 3× a day, with meals
	Milk thistle extract or silimarin tablets
	Herbal liver formulas (see Chapter 8)

Remarks Pumpkin, dark leafy greens, carrots and green food are packed with organic carotenes, which are essential for detoxifying and repairing the liver. Beetroot juice, milk thistle and dandelion all help detoxify and rebuild liver tissue. Since the liver filters the blood, a toxic liver means a toxic bloodstream and vice versa, so both must be cleansed together. Black grapes help clean both the bloodstream and the liver, especially if the skins and seeds are chewed very well and eaten together with the pulp. The chlorophyll in green food purifies blood and increases its capacity to carry oxygen, while bentonite molecules actively adsorb any toxins floating in the bloodstream and transport them to the kidneys for excretion. Liquorice and chrysanthemum tea detoxify and cool both the blood and the liver, and other herbal formulas may be included to amplify this effect.

CHAPTER 6

The 'Fast Lane': Fasting and Colonic Irrigation

Fasting is a perfect example of the hidden powers of nature that awaken when the ancient Taoist principle of *wu-wei*, 'not-doing' or 'non-interference', is put into practice. 'By doing nothing,' notes the *Tao Teh Ching*, 'the sage accomplishes everything.' In dietary terms, 'doing nothing' means eating nothing and letting nature take its course, and this abstinence awakens the body's most powerful cleansing and healing responses.

Fasting is nature's way of curing disease, restoring health and prolonging life. As all zookeepers and pet owners know, animals of every species instinctively refuse to eat when they are sick, and the same rule applies to animals in the wilderness. Long ago, humans also shared this natural revival instinct, and even today, primitive tribes in remote regions of Africa, Asia and the Amazon still have special 'sick houses' located on the outskirts of their villages, where the sick rest quietly and comfortably, without eating any food, for as long as it takes to recover their health.

Today, however, therapeutic fasting is dismissed by main-stream modern medicine as 'primitive'. As a prominent surgeon in New York once told this writer, 'Fasting went out with the horse-and-buggy!' Nevertheless, owing to the pioneering work of a few courageous health professionals during the latter half of the 20th century, the Western world has rediscovered the profound healing powers of fasting, and practitioners of alternative medicine are now applying it with success for conditions in which all other treatments fail. Moreover, recent scienctific research backed by extensive clinical studies has established conclusive proof that periodic fasting and calorie restriction are the one and only proven way to significantly extend lifespan.

On 28 May 1986, the Associated Press reported as follows regarding the results of a scientific study on ageing conducted in America, in which laboratory rats were periodically put on forced fasts:

> When the diets of laboratory rats are severely restricted, they live *far longer* than do otherwise identical animals that are allowed to eat as much as they want. In fact, researchers say such food limits are the *only way* they know of significantly extending these rodents' normal lifespans.

More recently, Dr Roy Walford, who was a member of the team that lived for two years in the experimental Biosphere project in America, has conducted even more exhaustive research on the link between calorie restriction and lifespan, using a variety of different species for his studies, including rats and dogs. In his book *Beyond the 120 Year Diet*, he presents his evidence, and it clearly demonstrates that calorie restriction prolongs the lifespan of all species tested by a factor of 50–80 per cent. In human terms, that would mean a lifespan of 120–150 years.

While long-term human studies on the effects of fasting on longevity have not yet been concluded, individual examples of several contemporary practitioners of therapeutic fasting are highly inspiring and most encouraging. Dr Norman Walker, for example, who advocated periodic fasting and daily consumption of raw juices, and practised what he preached, lived to the ripe age of 116, remaining active until the very end. Paul Bragg, who fasted for ten days four times a year for most of his life, lived almost as long as Dr Walker, and he too stayed healthy and productive until his final days. V. E. Irons, who cured himself of an 'incurable' crippling disease by fasting, then went on to develop the most efficient do-it-yourself fasting and internal cleansing system available today, would no doubt have lived a 'normal' human lifespan of 120, if fate had not intervened with a car accident at the age of 98. Each of these individuals, and others like them, rediscovered through their own experience what all animals and primitive tribesmen still know: that fasting is nature's way of cleansing and healing the body and regenerating the life force.

Abstaining from food permits the body's innate detox mechanisms to function at full capcity and allows immune responses to operate in high gear. When fasting, all of the energy and enzyme power that the body must normally use to digest and process food is diverted instead to 'digest disease', while the digestive system produces no new wastes in the body. Fasting also triggers the production of human growth hormone in the pituitary gland and releases it into the bloodstream, where it circulates throughout the body to repair damaged tissues, regenerate vital functions and rejuvenate the whole system. Normally, the production of growth hormone diminishes rapidly after humans reach adulthood, and the ever dwindling supply of this powerful regenerative hormone is one of the primary causes of ageing and the onset of chronic degenerative conditions. By stimulating secretion of human growth hormone, fasting not only helps cure disease and repair the body, it also slows down the ageing process, restores flagging vitality and prolongs life.

The cure of the sages

Fasting is not new. Hindu yogis, Buddhist monks and Taoist hermits have been fasting for thousands of years to enhance their vitality and extend their lifespans. A few years ago in India, an elderly meditation master set a world record by fasting non-stop for 200 days, during which time he took nothing whatsoever but plain water. Plato, Aristotle and other Greek philosophers whose thoughts laid the foundations of Western civilization fasted regularly to improve their physical health and sharpen their mental powers, and Pythagoras required all of his senior students to fast for 40 days as a means of purifying their bodies and minds prior to receiving his highest teachings. Practitioners of traditional medicine in ancient China also understood the direct link between human disease and the toxic filth that accumulates in the bowels as a result of unnatural eating habits. The Sung Dynasty physician Chang Tsung-cheng observed, 'If the stomach and bowels are blocked, then blood and energy stagnate.' While centuries ago the famous Chinese doctor, Chai Yu-hua, wrote 'Purging the bowels eliminates the source of poison, thereby permitting blood and energy to regenerate naturally. By cleaning the bowels we repair the body.'

The Bible mentions fasting 74 times, and Jesus himself fasted frequently, sometimes for as long as 40 days. When the Dead Sea Scrolls were unearthed in Palestine in the early 20th century, a most remarkable document written in Aramaic and dating from the 3rd century AD came to light. Translated into English in 1937 by Edmond Szekely under the title *The Essene Gospel of Peace*, this ancient text recounts in detail some of the most important healing work performed by Jesus among the people of Palestine, and much of it sounds very similar to what Dr Bernard Jensen writes about fasting and colonic irrigation in his book *Tissue Cleansing Through Bowel Management*. Unfortunately, none of this information ever found its way into the Bible, despite the fact that this gospel was recorded several hundred years earlier than other gospels that appear in the Bible. Perhaps the early editors of the Bible found the topic of colonic irrigation to be of too delicate a nature for inclusion in the Christian scriptures, but

since this ancient historical document contains teachings of vital
significance to the health of the Western world today, let's take
a quick look at some key passages and listen to what Jesus said
to his followers on the subject of detox and human health:

> Renew yourselves and fast. . . . Seek the fresh air of
> the forest and of the fields, and there in the midst of
> them shall you find the angel of air. . . . Then breathe
> long and deeply, that the angel of air may be brought
> within you. I tell you truly, the angel of air shall cast
> out of your body all uncleannesses which defiled it
> without and within . . .
>
> After the angel of air, seek the angel of water . . .
> Think not that it is sufficient that the angel of water
> embrace you outwards only. I tell you truly, the
> uncleanness within is greater by much than the
> uncleanness without. . . . Seek, therefore, a large trailing
> gourd, having a stalk the length of a man; take out its
> inwards and fill it with water from the river which the
> sun has warmed. Hang it upon the branch of a tree,
> and kneel upon the ground . . . and suffer the end of
> the stalk of the trailing gourd to enter your hinder
> parts, that the water may flow through all your bowels
> . . . . Then let the water run out from your body, that
> it may carry away from within it all the unclean and
> evil-smelling things. . . . And you shall see with your
> eyes and smell with your nose all the abominations
> and uncleannesses which defiled the temple of your
> body . . . . Renew your baptizing with water every day
> of your fast, till the day when you see that the water
> which flows out of you is as pure as the river's foam.

This method of cleansing and healing the body by means of
colonic irrigation using a trailing gourd and warm river water

was commonly practised among the ancient Essenes, among whom Jesus lived and studied during his early formative years, and it constitutes one of his most beneficial teachings for the welfare of humanity. Unfortunately, since all mention of this period in Jesus' life was deliberately excluded from the New Testament, this aspect of his work remains virtually unknown among Christians today, although it was common knowledge to Jesus' own disciples. The sages of the ancient world were well aware of the inseparable link between the state of the body and the state of the mind, for they knew that toxic blood and tissues form a breeding ground not only for disease and degeneration of the human body but also for the darkening and degradation of the human spirit. They knew the law that modern physicians and philosophers alike have forgotten: that whatever pollutes the body also pollutes the mind. That's why so many sacred scriptures of the ancient world prescribe fasting and detox as the first preliminary steps on the path of spiritual self-cultivation.

Today, the mutual dependence of physical and spiritual health has been largely forgotten, and few people see the causal connection between the massive pollution of the planet and degradation of the human body, and the rampant crime, chronic violence and spiritual malaise that marks human life in contemporary times. According to the psychophysiological prescription of the ancient sages who gave birth to Western civilization, cleaning up the planet and detoxifying the human body are the best medicine of all both for restoring peace on earth and reviving the health and spiritual integrity of humanity. It is only now, however, that scientific evidence validating the truth of this ancient teaching is beginning to emerge. In 1972, for example, the Moscow Research Institute of Psychiatry reported results of a clinical study in which fasting and tissue detox were successfully used, without recourse to any drugs whatsoever, to cure over 7,000 patients suffering from a variety of serious mental disorders that neither psychiatry nor drug therapy had helped in any way. This has since become known as the 'hunger cure' and is still practised in Russia.

Even a cursory glance at the current state of human affairs throughout the world today reveals two indisputable facts: one is that people everywhere and in all walks of life are getting sicker and more toxic than ever before in human history; the other is that human behaviour is growing more angry and violent, and world affairs are becoming more cruel and barbaric, day by day. Maybe it's already too late to take the slow lane of detox by gradual dietary reform; perhaps our only remaining hope is to take the plunge and leap directly into the 'fast lane' of detox by air and water alone.

The 'fast lane'

Tissue toxicity is a deadly serious condition, especially today, when so many carcinogens and other toxic chemicals contaminate our food and water and pollute the air we breathe. To give the reader an idea of just how serious the situation is, and what can be done about it, here's a graphic excerpt from the book *Detox Diet and Wellness Lifestyle*, by Dr Grady Deal, who operates a detox clinic in Hawaii:

> You may be unaware that the colon remains chronically impacted with accumulated faces and mucus backed all the way up to the small intestine . . . . In effect, your intestinal plumbing . . . backs up like a full and over-flowing septic tank. The blood vessels and lymph vessels in the colon pick up the toxins and carry them to all parts of the body . . . . The bloodstream becomes increasingly filled to overflowing with disease organisms . . . and toxins, where they circulate around the body, causing inflammation, water retention, weight

gain, irritation, corrosion, damage and disease. Faeces and toxins abnormally recirculated in the bloodstream as a result of chronic constipation explains why the eliminative organs of the skin and lungs have a strangely familiar unpleasant odour . . . in the form of smelly sweat . . . and bad breath that smells like faeces . . . . As a protective measure to get the disease-causing toxins out of circulation, the body removes these poisons from the bloodstream and stores them in cells and tissues, out of the way . . . causing what Dr Norman Walker calls tissue constipation, meaning the tissues are burdened with excess toxins which then cause cellular and tissue inflammation, congestion, eruptions, and disease. In general, excess toxins are continually stored in the cells [and] tissues . . . as long as the person is taking in that particular offending unhealthy food, allergen, drug, etc. When that specific food or substance is completely eliminated from the diet, only then do the cells eliminate that particular toxin from the cells back into the bloodstream and lymph on its way to the eliminative organs and out of the body. Once back in the bloodstream and lymph, the toxin does its dirty work of inflaming and irritating the body until it is eliminated and out of the body. This aggravation or worsening of symptoms is called a healing crisis. The person detoxifying from a toxin may get worse before they get better and they tend to crave the very food or habit which made him toxic initially.

Fasting is the fastest and most effective way to deal with this sort of blood and tissue toxicity, and to rid the body of the toxic residues and putrefactive wastes in the colon that continuously poison the bloodstream, clog the cells and sap vitality. Until these toxins are eliminated, there's simply no way that the body can repair and rebalance itself. Although there are milder methods of detox than fasting, they all take much longer and work less effectively, and none can match the deep healing power and life-prolonging benefits of fasting.

In order to gain those benefits, one must be willing to tolerate the unpleasant symptoms of the so-called 'healing crisis' that fasting always triggers after the third day. The healing crisis opens the gate to the state of radiant health and longevity that only fasting can create, and the discomfort of detox is the price one pays to pass through that gateway. The choice is yours: either you flush those poisons out of your system, or else you live with the consequences of retaining them for the rest of your life. As I note in my book *The Tao of Health, Sex & Longevity:*

> Unless you live an ascetic life far from civilization and avoid all dietary folly, your blood and other tissues are bound to accumulate toxins and gradually lose their functional vitality. If you don't purge yourself of these toxins on a regular basis, toxaemia gets worse and worse, until the body cannot stand it any longer and either purges itself spontaneously in the form of diarrhoea, acne, pimples, boils, 'liver spots', foul perspiration, body odour, bad breath and so forth, or else it simply gives up the battle and succumbs to cancer, tuberculosis and other fatal conditions.

Mega-fasts, mini-fasts, and semi-fasts

There are many different types of therapeutic fasting programme with varying degrees of intensity and duration. The most intensive detox and swiftest healing results are produced by completely foodless fasts in which nothing but water and a few internal cleansing supplements such as psyllium and bentonite are used. Semi-fasts, using water and supplements, plus one type of vegetable or fruit juice to provide energy and nutrition are easier to tolerate, and they, too, provide excellent cleansing and healing results. The so-called 'grape cure', in which nothing but black grapes are eaten for periods of one week to a full month, also qualifies as a sort of semi-fast, and it's particularly effective for purifying the bloodstream, detoxifying the liver and correcting serious gastro-intestinal disorders.

In order to be effective for detoxifying the blood and tissues, a therapeutic fast must continue for a minimum of three full days. That's how long it takes for the body's internal cleansing and healing mechanisms to shift into full gear. However, three days is not long enough to totally purify the bloodstream and detoxify the internal organs, nor is it long enough to experience the so-called 'healing crisis' which normally occurs sometime between the third and fifth day of a fast. The healing crisis marks the point in a fast when tissue detox has reached its peak, and symptoms of the body's most serious conditions come out of hiding and begin to manifest. For example, in someone with arthritis, the healing crisis occurs when the deepest deposits of toxic residues are dislodged and drawn out of the joints, causing pain in the joints and connective tissues. For someone suffering from heavy liver toxicity, the healing crisis comes as the most poisonous substances are dissolved and eliminated from the tissues of the liver, bringing out all the unpleasant symptoms of liver toxaemia, such as overwhelming fatigue and listlessness, anger and irritability, yellow eyes and skin, foul breath and body odour, and throbbing pain in the liver itself. The good news is that this 'crisis' marks the mid-point from which the rest of the fast is all downhill. It means that the worst of the detox stage of the fast has passed, and that the healing stage is beginning. That's why it's called a 'healing' crisis. Unless you continue a fast long enough to 'hit the wall' and pass through the dark gate of the healing crisis to reach the sunny state of radiant health, you will not succeed in fully correcting the root causes of your ills. Three days is certainly sufficient, however, to achieve a major cleansing of the bowels and bloodstream, and to rebalance the internal organs and partially detoxify the tissues.

The ideal duration for a therapeutic detox fast is 7–10 days. That's because it takes precisely seven days to completely purify the bloodstream and cleanse the lymphatic system of all residual wastes. When the blood and lymph have been totally purfied, it means the whole body and all its parts are free of toxicity, because pure blood and clean lymph automatically cleanse the body and eliminate toxins from the tissues on a day-to-day basis. If you reform your eating habits and change your diet after a detox fast, your blood and lymph will be able to keep your tissues clean far longer than they would if you continue polluting yourself with wrong eating habits and wrong food choices. Eating properly also means you won't need to fast so often to rid yourself of putrefactive digestive wastes and metabolic toxins. Generally speaking, one 7–10-day detox fast each year, while taking care to control your diet in between, is usually sufficient to protect you from serious diseases such as cancer and arteriosclerosis, prevent the onset of common degenerative conditions such as arthritis and senility, and pave the path to a long and healthy life. Almost anyone is capable of completing a seven-day fast, but for those who have never tried it and worry about going that long without food, a few three-day mini-fasts may be tried first, as a sort of 'warm-up'. This is a good way to gain confidence and gradually work up to a full seven-day fast.

The longest therapeutic detox fast known to this writer is the remarkable Breuss Cancer Cure, developed by the Austrian naturopath Rudolf Breuss. This involves a 42-day (6-week) fast during which only one cup of Breuss Vegetable Juice (fresh or bottled) is taken per day, sipped slowly by the teaspoonful, in addition to sage tea and one or two other herbal teas, depending upon the organs and tissues that need primary attention. While this may sound extreme, bear in mind that cancer is a serious condition that can easily kill the patient, and that the conventional therapies applied to cancer today, such as chemotherapy and radiation, are far more extreme in terms of the damage they do to the body than even the longest fast. In fact, mainstream cancer therapy often kills the patient faster than the cancer itself. On the other hand, no one has yet died as a result of trying the Breuss cancer cure, and to date there have been over 40,000 documented cases of cures for various forms of cancer, some of them already in the advanced stage of development, achieved by this method. Strangely, most people with cancer would rather submit to instant chemo or radiation therapy, despite their terrible side effects and dubious results, than endure a 42-day detox fast that has a proven track record as a real cure. It's hard to say whether their reluctance to try the fasting cure is due to lack of confidence in the method, or sheer fear of fasting.

The Breuss cancer cure is not only for treating cancer. As noted earlier, cancer is the final stage of tissue toxicity, and chronic tissue toxicity is the root cause of cancer. Therefore, the Breuss fasting programme may be used in shortened versions as a means of periodic cleansing general tissue detox, and this serves as very effective preventive therapy against the development of cancer. Unless you already have cancer and wish to use this method as a cure, it's not necessary to follow the Breuss fasting programme for the full 42 days. One to three weeks suffices to effectively detoxify the whole body.

Mini-fasts are those of less than three days. While these are not effective for serious detox purposes, they are an excellent form of maintenance between longer therapeutic fasts. For example, some people fast for one full day every week, taking nothing but pure water or one variety of alkalizing fruit or vegetable juice. This gives the digestive system a weekly rest, and allows the body a brief break from 'active duty' to readjust and rebalance itself. Another way is to fast for a period of two or three days each month, which has similar benefits to a weekly one-day fast. While mini-fasts do not provide the dramatic cleansing results of longer fasts, they are still quite effective as a form of regular preventive medicine against a wide range of diseases and degenerative conditions, especially if you do longer detox fasts from time to time. As the Greek writer Plutarch suggested, 'instead of medicine, fast for a day.'

Fasting supplements

Water is the primary cleansing agent involved in therapeutic fasting, and it's very important to drink at least 2 litres of purified alkaline water throughout the duration of any fast, even if you're using raw juices as well. In addition to water, a variety of very effective fasting supplements may also be utilized to amplify and accelerate blood purification and tissue detox, and to promote rapid healing during the course of a fast. These supplements are the 'tools of the trade' for the theaputic faster:

Psyllium This is the single most important supplement for cleaning and clearing the digestive tract, particularly the lower bowels. Its mucilaginous bulking properties also help curb hunger by making the stomach and intestines feel full.

Bentonite Colloidal bentonite acts like a 'magnetic mop' to neutralize and carry away toxins loosened from the bowel walls by the psyllium fibre. Five hundred times smaller than water molecules, the negatively charged micro-molecules of bentonite also enter the bloodstream and cellular fluids, where they latch onto positively charged toxins up to 200 times heavier and escort them through the bloodstream to the kidneys for excretion.

Green food Green food is by far the best nutritional supplement to use during a therapeutic fast. One of the richest and purest sources of blood-cleansing chlorophyll and life-sustaining nutrients, green foods are easy to assimilate and do not require complex digestion. They also provide sufficient metabolic energy to help counteract the food cravings that often arise while fasting.

Lemon juice During a fast, fresh lemon juice may be used to assist the detox process with its swift alkalizing and cleansing properties. As the only anionic (negative-ion charged) food source, it provides potent antioxidant activity and energizes the detox process. Lemon juice has natural affinity for the liver and stimulates bile production, thereby helping to detoxify and repair the liver. Thirty to 50 millilitres of fresh lemon juice may be added to the water when shaking up a dose of psyllium powder, in order to improve the rather dreary taste of the psyllium and enhance its cleansing properties.

Lactobacteria These are the so-called 'friendly flora' of the bowels, and they constitute one of the most important elements required for proper digestion of food, assimilation of nutrients and processing of digestive wastes. In healthy bowels, friendly bacteria should constitute about 80 per cent of total bacteria population, with putrefactive bacteria accounting for the remaining 20 per cent. In toxic bowels, such as those in over 95 per cent of the people on the planet today, the ratio is reversed, with putrefactive bacteria occupying 80 per cent or more of the bowel terrain, and the 'good guys' hanging on for dear life in ever dwindling numbers. A primary goal of any therapeutic fast is to completely dredge the bowels of *all* bacterial colonies, and to eliminate the septic filth in which they breed, then replenish the entire intestinal tract with fresh colonies of friendly lactobacteria. Psyllium and bentonite do the job of dredging out the old stuff very well, but it's up to you to take measures to introduce new colonies of beneficial lactobateria into the bowels after each fast, before the 'bad guys' sneak back in with ordinary food and take over again.

One way to replenish the bowels with friendly bacteria is to take a good lactobacteria supplement such as acidopholus, bifudus and other similar cultures used to make yoghurt. These come in powdered and capsule form, but you must be careful to purchase a reliable brand that retains its potency on the shelf.

Most brands on the market today contain virtually no living cultures. Another option is to eat fresh goat's milk yoghurt for about a week immediately after a fast, but this is not as effective as a high potency powdered supplement, because milk products produce mucus in the bowels, and it's best not to consume mucus-forming foods until after you've firmly established a new colony of friendly flora in your colon.

There's also a third way, one that you can easily prepare at home in your own kitchen. Popularly known as 'rejuvelac', fermented cabbage juice is one of the purest and most abundant sources of rejuvenating lactobacteria for the human digestive tract, and it does not require the use of any dairy products. After making the first batch, which takes about three days, each subsequent batch ferments quickly overnight by adding half a cup or so (100 ml) of the previous batch as a starter to prepare the next one. You may therefore keep the culture going day by day for as long as you wish, simply by chopping some cabbage, adding water and some starter from the last batch, and setting it aside to ferment for a day. A recipe for making your own rejuvelac at home is listed in the Recipes and Formulas section on page 328.

Regardless of whether you use dairy-based lactobacteria or cabbage rejuvelac, you should start taking it shortly before your first food when breaking a fast, and continue using it twice a day for at least ten days in order to ensure that a new colony of friendly bacteria establishes itself firmly in your bowels. Thereafter, it's a good idea to repeat this regimen several times each year, even without fasting first, in order to assist the friendly bacterial allies in your bowels to flourish and keep the putrefactive enemy under control.

Taking the plunge

While fasting for seven days completely purifies the bloodstream, cleanses the lymphatic system and detoxifies the tissues, fasting by itself will not remove the 2–7 kg of tough, toxic, mucoid matter that becomes deeply impacted in the bowels from years of wrong eating habits and wrong food choices that begin in childhood. The only way to rid your bowels of this rubbery toxic sludge is to dredge it out with a series of colonic irrigations done in conjunction with a therapeutic fast.

A hundred years ago, when pneumonia was still the leading cause of death in America, Dr J. H. Tilden of Denver, Colorado, cured thousands of people of this deadly disease, without ever losing a single patient, simply by treating them with fasting and colonic irrigation and nothing else, then putting them on a strict diet of fresh raw foods consisting mostly of fruit and vegetables. After decades of dependence on antibiotics, pneumonia has grown resistant to drug therapy and has once again become a major killer throughout the world. As with most infectious diseases, the real cure for pneumonia is not a new drug; it's an ancient naturopathic method that long pre-dates allopathic medicine, but has lain buried and unnoticed for centuries in the archives of medical literature. That method is fasting and colonic cleansing.

One man who, back in 1935, went to the library in search of a better cure and thereby rediscovered the curative powers of fasting and colonic irrigation, was V. E. Irons, an ordinary American businessman who, at the age of 40, had been diagnosed with a crippling arthritic spinal ailment called ankylosing spondylosis. His doctors told him that it was incurable and that he would soon be confined to a wheelchair. Refusing to accept their verdict, Irons began to study the medical literature recorded by such early luminaries of naturopathic medicine in America as Dr Tilden, Dr Kellogg and others, then decided to take matters into his own hands by treating his condition with a series of therapeutic fasts and self-administered colonics. The effect was almost immediate:

Within two months I had no more pain from displacement and within 14 months practically no spurs. All done with cleansing, fasting and natural foods – no drugs!

His experience, and the complete cure it effected, impressed him so deeply that he devoted the rest of his long life to research and development of this natural way to detoxify and heal the human body. In the process, he created a line of products that enables anyone to practise this powerful self-healing therapy safely and effectively at home. During the 1950s, V. E. Irons was briefly imprisoned in America for publicly stating his revolutionary views on human health and healing and refusing to recant them under legal pressure from the American medical establishment. Thirty years later, in an ironic turn of events that must have amused Irons, President Reagan heaped public praise on V. E. Irons for his excellent work in health and healing, and presented him with a national award for his contributions to the science of longevity. Irons remained healthy and active throughout the 98 years of his life, starting a second family at the age of 72 and fathering his last child at the age of 80.

During the course of his life, V. E. Irons perfected a system of self-detoxification based on fasting and colonic cleansing that this writer regards as one of the most important contributions

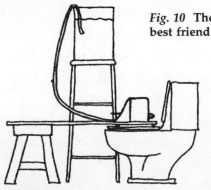

Fig. 10 **The 'Colema Board': the bowel's best friend**

to modern medicine and world health in the 20th century. In addition to his line of Vit-ra-tox internal cleansing supplements, Irons played a key role in the invention and development of the Colema Board (Fig. 10) – the bowel's 'best friend' and an indispensable tool for doing colonics yourself at home. Operated entirely by gravity, the Colema Board allows virtually anyone to safely administer their own colonic irrigations in the privacy of their own bathroom. As Irons notes in an interview, it's so easy that even a child can do it:

> My seven-year old son Robert frequently takes home colonics – all by himself. I'm 87 and I take them all the time. So, if you're anywhere between the ages of seven and 87, you should have no problems . . . . It is completely safe.

And yet, while people today don't hesitate to discuss the most intimate details of their – and others' – personal sex lives, the moment the world colon or bowel crops up in conversation, everyone winces uncomfortably and looks away, quickly changing the subject. Suggest that their bowels are bursting at the seams with mounds of foul putrefactive filth and that it might be a good idea for them to flush it all out with a series of colonics, and most people leap to their feet and start looking for the nearest exit. Here's what Irons has to say about such 'colonic cry-babies' in an interview he gave in 1982:

> If people can't take a simple home colonic to clean out their clogged, constipated, putrid colons, then tell them to start looking for an old rocking chair and cane . . . . If these people are afraid of all the 'horrors' that may happen to them when they stick a tiny plastic tube one 'micro-inch' up their fanny, there is just not much hope for them . . . . Many people will easily talk about the

most intimate sexual experiences – but by golly, they
will revolt at the first thought of discussing the colon.

Some people claim that fasting and raw juice therapy alone
can remove the hardened mucoid plaque from the colon wall,
but they are mistaken. Irons replies to this claim by saying,
'Forget it! It won't work . . . You must use the Colema Board
together with the intestinal cleansers, if you really want to
cleanse your colon properly. If you don't, the thick mucus
coating on the intestinal wall will never come off. It will stay
there till you die.'

It's important to remember that this tough toxic layer of putri-
fied mucus and partially digested protein was put there by you,
not by mother nature, as a result of your own unnatural eating
habits and food choices. Your body's natural cleansing mechanisms are not designed to deal with this unnatural mess; it
requires special methods to eliminate it. Those methods are
fasting and colonic cleansing, and anyone with the pluck to take
the plunge *always* gets spectacular results and *never* regrets the
decision to do it. Read V. E. Irons' description of what happens
when you include colonic irrigations in a therapeutic fast, based
on some of the cases he personally handled:

> You'll get fabulous results. Some of the worst smelling
> material known to man comes out when people do
> the programme right . . . . One woman passed more
> than a quart [1 litre] of black, vomitus, putrid mate-
> rial for three days in a row. One man passed a whole
> lot of material that looked like afterbirth. One man I
> know recently passed fourteen pounds [6.35 kg] of
> rotting material – all in one treatment . . . Just about
> everyone should get a lot of black, hardened mucus
> on about the fourth or fifth day, if he takes two five-
> gallon [19-litre] colonics a day . . . . Most of this mucus

is as black as charcoal and so tough you can't even cut it with a knife. In many cases, it's as tough as the rubber tubing of a bicycle tyre . . . . The longest we have had is 27 feet [8.2 m], in one piece. Sometimes it will come out as a pile weighing as much as 11 pounds [5 kg] and continuing to come out for several days to a week.

Despite clear evidence, most people these days, when told by a naturopath that their worst chronic ailments are caused by the seepage of poisons into the bloodstream from clogged, toxic bowels, and that they need a series of colonic irrigations to cure themselves, react with disbelief and reply defensively, 'Who, *me?*' The answer to that question is a resounding, 'Yes, *you!*' Thirty years ago, in a rare moment of candour, public health authorities in America acknowledged that 'over 90 per cent' of all Americans are running around with seriously clogged colons, such as those depicted in Fig. 11. Even longer ago, at the turn of the 20th century, the famous naturopath and highly respected surgeon Dr Harvey Kellogg said, 'Of the 22,000 operations I have personally performed, I have never found a single normal colon.' If that's the way it was a hundred years ago, it boggles the mind to imagine what a century of junk food, synthetic additives, chemically contaminated beef and dairy products, frozen pizzas and now genetically modified 'Frankinfood', have done to the contemporary Western colon. As Irons puts it, 'Regardless of your financial standing, regardless of your past health history, regardless of your age or sex, *YOU* do have this hardened mucus in your colon, and you will be amazed by what comes out of you.'

The only way to find out what comes out of you and to get rid of it once and for all is to climb aboard the 'Colema express' for a seven-day adventure of fasting and colonic irrigation.

Seven days aboard the Colema express

The seven-day fast and internal cleansing programme using Vit-ra-tox supplements and the Colema Board is V. E. Irons' great gift to the science of health and longevity, and today his family in California continues to produce and distribute this fine line of products and to provide printed information regarding the programme to anyone who requests it. Those interested in obtaining further information or ordering the products may do so by contacting the address given in the Mail-order Suppliers section on page 337.

To give the reader an idea of what to expect on a seven-day cleansing fast using detox supplements and colonics, here's a day-by-day description, based on personal experience, of a week on the Colema express – the fast lane to health, longevity and a squeaky clean colon:

Day 1 It's best to skip dinner the night before starting a thera-peutic fast, or to just eat fresh fruit, and to take 2–3 Vit-ra-tox

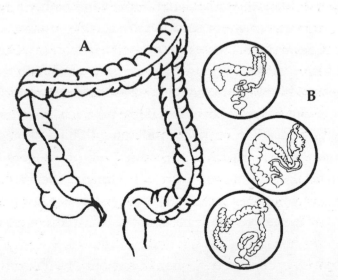

Fig. 11 **Clogged plumbing: the colon is the most 'out of shape' organ of all today**
A. Healthy colon as depicted in anatomy books
B. X-ray profiles of typical human colons today

herbal laxatives before bed, so that you begin the first day of the fast by completely evacuating the bowels of all residual faeces. In the morning, start taking the psyllium and bentonite cleansers, as well as the Greenlife and other nutritional supplements, according to the schedule outlined in the programme brochure, and take two 19-litre colonics per day. The first day is very easy and causes no discomfort, because the body's detox mechanisms have not yet reached high gear, and the tissues have not yet begun to discharge their toxins into the bloodstream.

Day 2 Continue taking the supplements and colonics. By mid-afternoon, you will probably begin to feel a bit weak and wobbly, tired and listless. This is *not* due to starvation or lack of nutrition. It's due entirely to the onset of the detox process, which switches on about 36 hours after you stop eating food. Digestive enzymes normally engaged in the endless task of digesting food in the stomach now enter the bloodstream instead and patrol the body on 'search and destroy' missions, dismantling damaged and cancerous cells, killing bacteria and viruses, and dissolving toxic deposits in the joints, organs and other tissues. All of these toxic wastes are then dumped into the bloodstream for excretion. For the first few days, the toxins come pouring out of the tissues much faster than the kidneys and skin can excrete them, leaving a backlog of toxic residues floating in the bloodstream. These toxins circulate around the body and through the brain while waiting to be eliminated, like aircraft circling an airfield while waiting their turn to land, and they can cause headaches, body pain, fatigue and irritability. You may, perhaps, derive a small measure of comfort from the knowledge that the worse you feel, the better the programme is working for you to detoxify and heal your body, and that it will all pass in a few more days. There is no shortcut to bypass the symptomatic discomforts of detox, although you may lessen them with herbal teas, hot mineral baths, massage and other methods such as infra-red sauna. There's always a certain degree of 'no pain, no gain' dynamics when it comes to detox. But with fasting, the gain is so much greater and lasts so much longer than the temporary discomfort it causes, that it seems a negligible price to pay for the benefits.

Day 3 The detox process continues to accelerate and intensify today, making you feel even more tired and uncomfortable. If you feel particularly low, you may take a few extra doses of bentonite, which helps neutralize the toxic overload in the bloodstream. You may also take some extra Greenlife to increase the blood's capacity to carry oxygen and provide additional fuel for metabolic energy. This is the day that you start to approach the threshold of the healing crisis, which marks the peak intensity of the detox phase and the beginning of the healing process. It's no coincidence that this is also the day that first-time fasters start to waver and toy with the idea of terminating the fast. Do *not* surrender to that temptation! You've already come this far, and you'll regret it if you deprive yourself of the final rewards of the fast by quitting now.

Day 4 For most people, this is the most difficult day, especially if they are highly toxic, because this is the day that the healing crisis usually occurs. The body excretes a foul odour and clammy sweat, the breath stinks of rotting sewage, and the tongue fur gets coated with white and yellow slime. All of this is toxic waste from the deepest tissues of the body coming to the surface for elimination, and it's always a sign of successful detox. Don't give up now! This is the halfway mark, and if you can make it through to the end of the day, the rest is all downhill, and you will easily finish the programme.

Day 5 Depending upon how toxic you were to begin with, the healing crisis will either pass today, or continue with ever diminishing intensity until the next morning. Either way, you will start feeling better today, and since the heaviest toxins are out, your body will have a lot more energy to spare for ordinary functions. You'll start to notice a lightness in your limbs, a supple flexibility in your joints, and a rapidly growing clarity and joy in your mind. You will realize from the way you feel on this day, without a shadow of doubt, that you are in the midst of the most profound cleansing and healing experience of your life, and that what you are doing is the best possible way to repair your body, preserve your health and prolong your lifespan. That insight alone usually suffices to carry you through to the end of the programme.

Day 6 Energy returns rapidly now, and the blood and tissues are almost completely purified. Your body has already begun to replace damaged cells, rebuild blood and repair organs and tissues; as a result, you feel yourself growing stronger by the hour, even though you have not eaten any food for nearly a week. You should continue taking two colonics per day, because the biggest amounts of the most deeply impacted mucoid matter and putrefactive waste are flushed out of the colon on the last two or three days of the fast, after the superficial layers of sludge have been removed. As Irons and anyone else who has ever done this programme remark, 'You will be amazed by what comes out of you', especially in the last few days, after not eating anything for nearly a week.

Day 7: By now, you should feel healthier, and more energized and well balanced than you can ever remember feeling before, and you probably won't feel much hunger for food. Many people feel as though they could easily fast for a few more days, and indeed you could, if you wish. Recalling the heavy heaps of putrid waste matter that poured out of your bowels, and realizing how much better you feel after ridding your body of this toxic load, you will probably resolve to change your diet and eating habits in order to avoid polluting your bowels, blood and bodily tissues again with wrong food choices, indigestible food combinations and chemical contaminants. Don't forget to take a good lactobacteria supplement for a week or two after any fast, and be sure to break your fast gradually and carefully by eating only fresh fruits and vegetables for a day or two, then slowly returning to a normal daily diet of wholesome natural foods properly prepared and correctly combined.

Try taking the Colema express. You probably won't like the ride very much, but you'll love the results!

CHAPTER 7

'The Angel of Sunlight': Heliotherapy

Ancient Chinese medical texts describe sunlight as a form of 'nourishment for the brain', and the prescription they give to correct conditions caused by deficiency of this vital 'nutrient' is to 'administer sunbeams' to the patient's eyes and skin. These texts clearly state that 'sunlight benefits the brain by stimulating production of vital essence'. In the brain, 'vital essence' refers to pituitary hormones and neurotransmitters.

Many ancient cultures understood the vital link between health and sunlight, and they knew that sunlight could be applied as a form of medicine to purify, heal and rebalance the human system. In *The Essene Gospel of Peace*, after teaching his followers how to cleanse their bodies internally with water, Jesus advises them as follows:

> Seek the angel of sunlight. Put off your shoes and your clothing and suffer the angel of sunlight to embrace all your body . . . that the angel of sunlight may be brought within you. And the angel of sunlight shall cast out of your body all evil-smelling and unclean things which defiled it without and within.

Modern medical science has unravelled the mystery of the mechanism whereby 'the angel of sunlight' casts out 'unclean things' from the human body. They call it the oculo-endocrine system, and the new branch of science spawned by this discovery is known as photobiology. The essential factor in sunlight that 'nourishes the brain' is the invisible band of long-wave ultra-violet (UV) light that enters the eye along with the visible frequencies of light. UV light has both long-wave and short-wave forms; it is only excessive exposure to the short-wave variety that damages the eyes and skin. Long-wave UV light, however, is an absolutely essential factor for sustaining human health; it can also be applied as a tool for detox and healing.

Here's how the oculo-endocrine system works: when natural, full-spectrum sunlight enters the eyes, the visible bands of light excite the cells in the retina known as rods and cones to produce the colours and forms of ordinary vision. The invisible long-wave UV frequencies, which hit the retina together with the visible bands, activate a special layer of cells in the retina called epithelial cells, which are designed by nature precisely for the purpose of receiving these invisible frequencies of ultraviolet light within the eyes. Long-wave UV stimulation to the epithelial cells in the retina produces a powerful neural pulse that is carried along the optic nerve and delivered directly to the pituitary and pineal glands, where these signals stimulate the production of essential hormones that regulate the entire endocrine system and thereby determine the strength and speed of the body's natural immune responses.

The pituitary plays a particularly important role in the ocular-endocrine system, especially for immune response. Known as the body's 'master gland', the pituitary secretes hormones that regulate and balance all the other glands in the endocrine system, and without sufficient stimulation from long-wave UV light via the retina and optic nerve, the pituitary is deprived of its most essential form of 'nourishment' and the entire oculo-endocrine system malfunctions, resulting in impaired immune response. With all the smog, smoke, dust, chemicals and other pollution in the air today, the strength and quality of sunlight reaching the earth has been seriously reduced, resulting in widespread UV deficiency and contributing to the overall deterioration in human immune response. The Smithsonian Institute reports a 15 per cent reduction in the overall intensity of sunlight reaching the earth over the past 75 years, with an even greater drop of 27 per cent in the UV part of the spectrum. This is causing problems for human health that are quite similar to the immuno-suppressive effects produced by polluted sources of food, water and air.

The biggest problem caused by sunlight deficiency is weak immune response and low resistance, which not only reduces the body's defence against disease and degeneration, but also erodes its ability to detoxify and repair itself. The effects of 'light pollution' on human health in big cities and heavily industrialized regions are similar to those of pollutants in food, water and air: they all fail to deliver the essential elements and energies required to sustain strong immunity and resistance. This problem is further aggravated by the sedentary, indoor lifestyles led by most people, which keeps them out of the sun all day long and almost always places a layer of glass between their eyes and sunlight whenever they do venture briefly outdoors.

All glass blocks out beneficial long-wave UV frequencies in sunlight. That means your oculo-endocrine system receives no nourishment and stimulation when you're sitting behind the windshield of a car, looking through a window in your home or office, riding on a bus or train, or walking in broad sunlight wearing any kind of eye glasses. Only plastic windowpanes and lenses allow beneficial UV waves to pass through and enter the eyes. Herein lies another contributing factor in the modern syndrome of chronic fatigue, ill health and mental malaise experienced by people who spend their entire working lives seated at desks in glass office towers, and most of their leisure time seated indoors at home watching TV in artificially lit homes. The net result of such light-deficient lifestyles is an acquired immune deficiency caused by chronic 'solar malnutrition' and the consequent imbalance in the oculo-endocrine system.

Let's look at a few concrete examples that illustrate this problem. During the Hong Kong flu epidemic that swept through America in the winter of 1968–69, entire factories and department stores in Sarasota County, Florida, were forced to close down due to the high incidence of flu among their employees. However, at one large factory where plastic windowpanes and full-spectrum indoor lighting had recently been installed, not a single employee fell ill during the entire duration of the epidemic. Similar results have since been observed in other places where full-spectrum light sources have been installed.

Another good example of how crucial the oculo-endocrine system is to human health is the situation in state schools in America and other 'advanced' nations. Severe hyperactivity, chronic violence, inability to concentrate and other behavioural problems have become so severe among young school children that many of them are now dosed daily with powerful sedatives, tranquillizers and amphetamines, which in turn lead to even more severe lifelong health problems, such as drug addiction and liver damage. However, when ordinary fluorescent lights, which have an extremely irritating effect on the oculo-endocrine system, were replaced with full-spectrum lighting and glass windowpanes were replaced with plastic in several selected school districts, these behavourial problems virtually vanished within a few weeks, and many 'problem children' were suddenly transformed into model students. Similarly positive results were observed in *every* classroom tested. Incredibly, this research has been deliberately ignored and suppressed owing to its implications for conventional indoor lighting systems everywhere.

A third example is the 'winter blues' syndrome that had long been observed in countries such as Sweden and Canada, where long winters and short days produce a critical deficiency in beneficial UV stimulation during that time of year. By mid-winter, these countries experienced a significant rise in deaths due to disease as well as suicide, and the reason turned out to be 'starvation' of the pituitary gland due to insufficient exposure to full-spectrum sunlight. Today, these countries have light clinics where people can go for their daily dose of long-wave UV light energy, and many homes, offices and public places use full-spectrum indoor lighting to compensate for the decrease in natural outdoor sources during the depths of winter.

'Skin deep'

Skin is the second important receptor for assimilating essential nourishment and energy from solar radiation. In 1967, a group of Russian scientists reported the results of extensive research in this field as follows:

> If human skin is not exposed to solar radiation (direct or scattered) for long periods of time, disturbances will occur in the physiological equilibrium of the human system. The result will be functional disorders of the nervous system and a vitamin-D deficiency, a weakening of the body's defences, and an aggravation of chronic diseases.

The main mechanism whereby sunlight provides essential 'nutrition' to the human body through exposure to skin is vitamin D production. Sunlight stimulates the tissues below the skin to produce vitamin D, which is an essential co-factor for the assimilation and utilization of calcium in the body. Without the presence of vitamin D, there's no way that the body can absorb even the purest, most potent sources of calcium, and without adequate supplies of calcium, there's no way the body can detoxify and repair itself. Solar deficiency is therefore a primary contributing factor to chronic calcium deficiency, and this in turn is one of the main reasons that modern humans, especially in urban areas, have such weak teeth and bones.

It's a fact of modern lifestyle that most people in the Western world do not get adequate exposure to clear, full-spectrum sunlight, and the few who do go out in the sun are like the proverbial 'mad dogs and Englishmen', tanning their hides in the noonday sun for cosmetic purposes only. This is an abuse of sunlight that's tantamount to gluttony in food. The proper daily 'dosage' for sunlight is about 30 minutes, more or less, and this should be administered only before 10:30 am or after 3:30 pm. As Dr Theodore Baroody states in his book *Alkalize or Die*, 'At least ½ to 1 hour of direct sunlight a day is requisite for the body's system to produce proper hormonal levels and assist alka-line-acid balances . . . . Between 11:00 am and 3:00 pm, the sun is too direct and produces an acid effect in the body through its radiations.' So here again we see how insufficient exposure to beneficial sunlight, as well as excessive exposure to damaging sunlight, contribute to the current crisis in human health. Not only does this problem produce critical imbalances in the oculo-endocrine system, it also has an acid-forming influence on the blood and other bodily fluids, which makes it a major contrib-uting factor to chronic acidosis and tissue toxaemia.

Heliotherapy for detox and healing

The therapeutic power of sunlight is another reason that health resorts and healing spas have traditionally been located by the sea or high up in the mountains. Like the high negative ion count in mountain and seaside air, the clear bright sunlight in such locations provides strong support for the many immune responses involved in detox and healing. By stimulating the pituitary gland via the oculo-endocrine system, sunlight assures an adequate daily supply of the essential hormones required to repair and rebalance the body. In addition, by prompting production of vitamin D, the essential co-factor required by the body to assimilate and utilize calcium, sunlight also assures the abundant supplies of calcium needed for detox and healing.

While it's definitely a big advantage to do a detox programme at a time and a place with lots of sunshine, you don't need to spend a fortune at a fancy spa to find good sunlight for a week or two. You can avoid the expense of staying in health resorts and spas by designing your own detox programme and doing it in a sunny time and place of your own choosing. If there is no sunny season where you live, or you cannot find sufficient peace and privacy at home, you may travel instead to the nearest mountains or seashore, rent an inexpensive room or cottage for a week or two, and do it yourself. You don't need luxury and fancy frills for a detox programme; what you need is peace of mind and plenty of personal privacy, clean air and pure water, and clear bright sunlight.

The best times of day for heliotherapy, or 'therapeutic sunbathing', are before 10:30 in the morning and after 3:30 in the afternoon, when the sun rides low in the sky and doesn't damage skin or eyes. Twenty to 30 minutes of exposure per session, and one or two sessions per day, are sufficient to achieve the desired therapeutic benefits, and total daily exposure should not exceed one hour. The more skin you expose while sunbathing, the greater the therapeutic benefits. This also applies to the eyes: don't wear sunglasses during heliotherapy, because they block out the beneficial long-wave UV frequencies in sunlight, and these are the solar factors which activate the ocular-endocrine system and elevate immune response.

Unfortunately, it's not always possible to find a sunny time and place to do a detox programme, especially if it's mid-winter in the northern latitudes and your finances are limited. Nevertheless, when the condition of your health demands that you 'clean up your act' and detoxify your system without delay, you may bring the healing power of natural sunlight into your own home by installing full-spectrum light bulbs and lighting systems, which are now widely available. Like food, water and air, modern technology has analyzed the 'active ingredients' in sunlight and developed 'solar supplements' to compensate for the degradation in the quality of natural sources of these essential elements for life. Much of this new light technology is based on the work of time-lapse photographer John Ott, who accidentally discovered the healing powers of sunlight when he stepped on his sunglasses and broke them while working on an outdoor project to film the growth cycles of plants. Too busy to buy new glasses, he worked without them, and a few weeks later he noticed that the painful arthritis he'd suffered for many years was disappearing fast. Subsequent research revealed that the UV light which his sunglasses had formerly blocked from entering his eyes, had relieved his arthritis by stimulating his pituitary to secrete the hormones that signal the adrenal glands to produce the natural steroids which constitute the body's own built-in remedy for this condition.

Today there is a wide range of full-spectrum lighting available on the market, including the Ott Light and the Ott Bulb, which produce indoor light containing the complete spectrum of natural light frequencies, both visible and invisible, found in clear bright sunlight. These light fixtures may be used in any home or office; you could even take your own full-spectrum light bulbs with you to a health resort or beach cottage, and use them to light your rooms there. In the absence of adequate sources of whole natural sunlight outdoors, full-spectrum lighting indoors provides all the essential frequencies of sunlight required to stimulate the oculo-endocrine system, thereby sustaining strong immune response and promoting production of vitamin D for calcium assimilation. Full-spectrum lighting is an excellent form of preventive medicine in daily life as well. By lighting your home and your place of work with 'whole light', you provide yourself with an additional line of defence against disease and degeneration, and help counteract the immuno-suppressive effects of harmful artificial light frequencies such as those produced by television screens and fluorescent lights.

Another form of indoor heliotherapy that has recently been developed is the infrared sauna. Unlike ordinary saunas, which heat the bodily tissues and induce perspiration by sheer force of heat, infrared saunas heat the deepest organs and tissues of the body by virtue of the radiant penetrating energy of the infrared band of natural light. This radiant energy heats the internal tissues without overheating the skin and respiratory system, as ordinary saunas often do. As it penetrates into the deeper, denser tissues below the skin, the infrared heat softens deposits of crystallized toxins and acid wastes in joints, nerves and connective tissues, allowing them to be dissolved, diluted and carried away for excretion via blood, lymph and sweat. Holistic healing centres and health spas are beginning to include infrared saunas among their therapeutic facilities, and there are also smaller units available for home installation.

'Let there be light'

In previous chapters, we've already seen how essential factors in food, water and air may be utilized as effective tools for detox, and now sunlight too may be added to our growing arsenal of weapons to do battle with tissue toxicity, strengthen immune defences and protect our health. Similarly, just as good food, pure water and clean air may be fully integrated into daily life as long-term defence against disease, degeneration and prema-ture demise, so full-spectrum light may also be relied upon as a daily source of life-supporting elements and energies. While getting adequate daily exposure of eyes and skin to natural sunlight outdoors is no doubt the best way to achieve this, in reality, most people are far too busy to take the time to do this on a daily basis, their schedules simply won't permit it, or else they live in places where the sun doesn't shine much.

If that's your situation, then you have two alternatives. If you live in sun-starved areas such as big cities or far northern latitudes where the winters are long and the days short, you can ensure there is light in your own home and office/shop/studio by using full-spectrum indoor lighting systems. Alternatively, if you live in a sunny region, you can 'harvest' sufficient long-wave UV radiation from the sun each day by quickly doing a simple set of eye exercises early in the morning or late in the afternoon. To do this, stand facing the sun anytime between sunrise and 8:30 am, or between 4:30 pm and sunset. Without looking directly at the sun, roll your eyes in big circles around the sun, so that sunlight bathes the entire surface of the retina. Roll 10–20 times in each direction. Then close your eyes while facing the sun and blink rapidly ten times, shut them again for a minute and blink rapidly another ten times. That's it: your pituitary gland has now received its daily dose of whole unrefined sunlight, and your endocrine system has received its solar tune up for the day. Go forth and shine!

CHAPTER 8

The Eliminators: Herbal Detox

Traditional herbal pharmacopoeia contain hundreds of medicinal herbs that effectively eliminate toxic substances and flush out residual metabolic wastes from the blood and tissues. They also help repair toxic damage to the organs and restore functional balance to the whole system. The great advantage of using natural herbs rather than chemical drugs to repair and rebalance the body is that each herb may be specifically selected to target particular organs and tissues with very precise and intensive detox therapy, without causing hazardous side effects in other parts of the body, as most chemical drugs do. Such therapeutic precision can only be achieved with medicines derived directly from nature by virtue of sympathetic resonance between their essential energies and similar organic energy frequencies in the body. Each and every herb has what TCM calls a 'natural affinity' (*gui jing*) for specific tissues and organ-energy systems in the body, and after many millenia of continuous clinical practice, traditional herbalists have determined the specific natural affinities and therapeutic actions of thousands of medicinal herbs. All of this knowledge has been carefully recorded and preserved for posterity in traditional herbal manuals that are still in use today, and it may easily be applied at home to produce swifter, deeper, more effective results in any detox programme.

Herbal supplements may be used to accelerate and amplify detox and healing in programmes based on detox diets, as well in fasting programmes. When using herbs for detox support in therapeutic fasting programmes, it's best to prepare them as whole herbal teas, which have gentler, less aggressive effects than concentrated herbal extracts. When fasting, the body becomes far more sensitive to the effects of all external supplements, and therefore a mild herbal tea delivers the same therapeutic potency to someone who's fasting, as a concentrated extract of the same herb would to someone on a detox diet, but without the intensity of condensed extracts. When used as supplements in a detox diet, herbs may be taken in all forms, from the mildest teas to the strongest tinctures, powders and tablets.

In traditional Chinese medicine, all herbs are categorized in two ways: according to their natural affinities for specific organs and tissues, which determines where in the body their therapeutic energies go; and according to the nature of their bio-active energies, which determines their therapeutic effects. The latter classification is based on the ancient Chinese theory of the five elemental energies (*wu hsing*), which in food and medicine manifests as the five essential flavours (*wu wei*). Most detox herbs in TCM belong to the 'bitter' category of medicines, and this also holds true in traditional Western herbalogy. No doubt this is the origin of the term 'bitter medicine', for prior to the advent of chemical drugs and artificially flavoured foods, most diseases were treated with cleansing bitter herbs and foods, and medicinal herbal 'bitters' were a common household item in homes throughout the world. Today, not only have insipid chemical pills replaced bitter herbal potions in medicine, widespread addiction to sugar has led to a 'sweet tooth' syndrome that has virtually eliminated bitter flavours from modern Western diets. And yet, according to the principles of traditional herbalogy, bitter flavours are nature's antidote for toxaemia, and bitter herbs and foods carry energies into the body that purify the blood-stream, detoxify the tissues and initiate healing responses.

Let's take a look at the major organs systems involved in the detox process, and see how medicinal herbs may be utilized to cleanse their tissues and rebalance their functions, while also protecting them from toxic damage during the detox process.

Liver: cleaning the filter

In TCM, the liver is described as the 'chief of staff' of the internal organs. It holds responsibility for filtering toxins from the blood, breaking down complex proteins, fats and carbohydrates, and providing the bloodstream with a constant infusion of nutrients for delivery to the various tissues of the body. External signs of internal liver toxicity include yellow eyes and blurry vision, brittle fingernails and cracked toenails, and the negative emotions of anger, depression and irritability. During detox, the liver must store an overload of toxic wastes discharged from the tissues, while the bloodstream gradually moves them out to the various excretory organs for elimination. Therefore, people with a history of liver toxicity, especially from excessive use of alcohol and drugs, or from chemical contamination, should include a few herbal liver cleansers among the supplements they select as supports for a detox programme.

The most effective herbs for detoxifying the liver are milk thistle and dandelion root, which may be taken as whole herbal teas, capsules of the ground powdered herbs or liquid extracts. Milk thistle has particularly potent liver cleansing properties. Its primary active ingredient is silymarin, a compound that has stronger antioxidant properties in the liver than vitamins E, C or betacarotene. Silymarin may be taken directly in tablet or capsule form, 100 mg three times a day, as liver support during detox. In addition to detoxifying the liver, milk thistle stimulates production of the proteins required to build new cells and repair damaged tissues in the liver. A formula for liver detox tea, in which milk thistle and dandelion are combined with four other herbal liver cleansers, is given in the Recipes and Formulas section on page 329. Dragon River Herbals (see Suppliers section) produces a formula called Rejuvenate Liver Regenerator, which is a pure, high-potency blend of extracts of dandelion, milk thistle, red clover, burdock and cleavers in concentrated liquid form. This is an excellent supplement to use for detoxifying and repairing the liver in conjunction with a detox diet of one to three weeks' duration.

A quick and easy way to give the liver a deep, intensive cleanse is to do the 'liver flush'. This may be done once a day for a period of three to ten days, preferably in the morning, as a means of flushing extra toxins from the liver during a detox diet programme, but it's not a suitable method to use while fasting. The liver flush prompts an intensive cleansing purge in the liver, and it's particularly beneficial in cases of long-term chronic liver toxicity. For best results, supplement the liver flush by drinking plenty of liver detox tea. Here's how to do it:

> Mix one cup (250 ml) of your choice of freshly squeezed citrus juices, such as orange and grapefruit, but be sure to include some fresh lemon juice. Add enough pure water to dilute it to taste. Add the juice of 2 cloves of garlic and ½ teaspoon of freshly grated ginger juice (grate the ginger, then squeeze the pulp through a cloth). Mix in 1 tablespoon high-grade virgin olive oil and ½ teaspoon cayenne, then shake it all together in a glass jar with a lid until well blended, and drink it down. Follow with one or two cups (250–500 ml) of liver detox tea, sipped slowly.

Although the liver flush includes two food items (lemon juice and olive oil), these are therapeutic foods with an affinity for the liver, and they work synergistically with the three active herbal ingredients – garlic, ginger and cayenne. Performed regularly once or twice a year, this is an excellent regimen for general liver maintenance and preventive protection against disease and degeneration there.

Chinese herbal medicine, which is renowned for the efficacy of its formulas for treating liver damage, offers some special high-potency liver detox formulas that may be used in cases of severe liver toxicity due to drug, alcohol or chemical poisoning. They may also be used to treat the various forms of hepatitis. These are powerful formulas with strong effects, and they should only be used within the context of an overall detox diet programme, preferably with the assistance of a health professional. In a previous title, *A Handbook of Chinese Healing Herbs*, I present a classic Chinese formula for healing severe liver damage that has demonstrated repeated efficacy in clinical practice. Known as Major Bupleurum with Artemisia Decoction, this formula is given in the Recipes and Formulas section on page 329, along with a few guidelines on diet and other factors that should be followed when using it.

Blood and lymph: the pipelines

In TCM, the condition of the bloodstream is regarded as a primary indicator of health and disease, and a decisive factor in healing. Blood is responsible for delivering oxygen and nutrients to the cells, and carrying away carbon dioxide and other metabolic wastes for excretion. In Chinese medicine, great emphasis is given to purifying the bloodstream as an essential preliminary step in curing any ailment. The lymph deals with the coarsest toxins and most highly acidic wastes in the body, and it plays an especially important role during detox, when the bloodstream becomes overloaded with toxic residues discharged from the tissues. Unlike blood, lymph does not have its own pump to move it through the system, as the heart pumps blood. Instead, lymph depends on the force of gravity and regular movements of the body for its mobility, which is why the lymphatic system becomes so vulnerable to stagnation in sedentary people.

Herbs which purify the blood and lymph are known as 'alternatives', because they alter the state of these vital bodily fluids from toxic to pure. The most widely used blood alternatives in Western herbalogy include echinacea, yerba mansa, chaparral, red clover, burdock and yarrow. These may be taken singly or in various combinations, either as whole teas, or concentrated tablets and extracts. A tasty tea used in TCM to detoxify and 'cool' the bloodstream is made by steeping dried chrysanthemum blossoms and liquorice root for 15–20 minutes in boiling hot water; this may be sipped throughout the day and night during any detox programme to help keep the bloodstream clean and prevent overheating of the blood due to toxic overload. Cayenne also helps cleanse the bloodstream during detox, by giving a strong boost to circulation and thereby accelerating delivery of toxins to the excretory organs for elimination.

An alterative formula that cleanses both the blood and the lymph may be prepared by combining equal amounts of concentrated liquid extracts of echinacea, red root, baptisia root, thuja leaf, stillingia root, blue flag root and prickly ash bark. Take 20–30 drops of this blend in warm water, 3–5 times a day, between meals. This treatment may be started during a detox programme, then continued for up to three more months, especially when deep tissue cleansing is required, or if the immune system is weak.

The most important herbs for cleansing lymph are red root, echinacea, ocotillo, red clover, cleavers, mullein, figwort, prickly ash and poke weed. As with blood alternatives, these may be taken singly or in various combinations, as teas, tablets or tinctures. Remember, however, that during a therapeutic detox fast, these herbs should only be used in the form of steeped or simmered teas, not concentrated extracts. A formula for lymphatic detox tea is given in the Recipes and Formulas section on page 331.

Kidneys and bladder

In TCM, the kidney system is referred to as the 'minister of power', and its energy is so essential that it's also known as the 'root of life'. One reason the kidney system is so important to overall health and vitality is that the adrenal glands are attached to the top of the kidneys. Therefore, whenever the kidneys become toxic or weak, the adrenal glands falter as well, weakening immune response as well as sexual potency. According to TCM, kidney-energy also regulates the condition of bone and marrow, which produces red and white blood cells. As a result, when kidney energy is deficient, blood becomes weak and immune response is impaired. The kidneys themselves are responsible for filtering the fluid wastes of metabolism from the bloodstream, and the bladder is the primary outlet for eliminating these acid wastes from the body. For those with deficient kidney function and adrenal insufficiency, it's a good idea to take some form of herbal kidney support during a detox programme, in order to protect the kidneys and bladder from toxic damage and assist them in excreting wastes quickly from the body.

An excellent formula for cleansing the kidneys and bladder and balancing kidney functions is Breuss kidney tea, which may be used in detox diets as well as during therapeutic fasts. You should start drinking this tea on the first day of a detox programme, and continue taking it three times a day for exactly three weeks, even if your detox programme is only for a few days. You may also use this herbal tea for three consecutive weeks, once or twice a year, in conjunction with your regular daily diet, as an effective means of periodic kidney cleansing and preventive protection against kidney disease. The formula for Breuss kidney tea is given in Recipes and Formulas on page 331. Another formula that's particularly effective for cleansing the urinary tract and bladder is given on page 332.

Parsley tea, which can easily be prepared in the kitchen from fresh or dried parsely leaf, has a strong affinity for the kidneys and is an excellent kidney cleanser. Parsley also soothes the kidney tissues when they become inflamed from passing too many toxins too fast during intensive detox, and since fresh parsley is readily available in most markets and many home gardens, it's a good idea to keep some on hand in the kitchen, in case you need to give your kidneys a refreshing flush during detox. To prepare a potent herbal kidney cleanser that contains parsley as well as herbs which strengthen the entire urinary system, combine equal amounts of finely ground powders of dried gravel root, juniper berries, hydrangea, uva ursi, parsley, marshmallow, bladderpod, ginger and burdock root. Take 1 level teaspoon of this powder three times a day, between meals, either in capsules or stirred into a cup of hot water. Powdered herbs generally have stronger, longer-lasting therapeutic effects than whole teas, but should not be used while fasting.

Bowels: dredging the sewer

Known in TCM as the 'minister of transport', the colon trans-forms digestive wastes from liquid into solid form, recovering and recyling most of the water and moving the solids onwards to the rectum for elimination. When the colon gets clogged with putrefactive wastes, toxic residues are diverted to the lungs and skin for excretion, causing lung congestion, bronchial infections and festering skin eruptions. Constipation and bowel toxicity are the primary causes of blood and tissue toxaemia throughout the body, because deeply impacted toxins in the colon constantly pass through the colon wall by osmosis and pollute the bloodstream. Of all the organs in the human body today, the lower bowel is by far the most congested with toxic waste, and dredging these poisonous wastes from the colon should be a primary goal of any detox programme. Unless the colon is thoroughly cleansed, no matter how well you clean your blood, liver and other tissues, they will all soon become polluted again by toxins seeping into the bloodstream from the colon.

In TCM, rhubarb is the sovereign remedy for constipation, and it may be used singly or in combination with other bowel cleansing herbs. A classic Chinese formula using rhubarb, which I listed in *A Handbook of Chinese Healing Herbs* as 'moisten bowel decoction', is given in the Recipes and Formulas section on page 333. The Vit-ra-tox line of internal cleansing supplements includes an excellent herbal laxative in convenient tablet form, containing cascara sagrada, aloe curacao and liquorice. This formula assists the elimination of impacted mucoid matter and putrefactive bacterial wastes in the colon, softens and clears solid obstructions which clog the bowels, and stimulates vigorous peristalsis in the large intestine. It may be ordered by mail directly from the source listed in the Suppliers section.

A very effective way to deal with chronic constipation and clear clogged bowels during a detox programme is to use powdered psyllium seed blended with various powdered herbs that have colon cleansing properties. Herbal Fibre Blend, made by AIM, has already been mentioned as an excellent example of this supplement. You can also prepare your own blend of psyllium and bowel detox herbs by combining 115 g ground psyllium with 1 level teaspoon each of the following powdered herbs: liquorice root, slippery elm, cascara sagrada and black walnut hulls. Mix together until well blended, and use the same way as plain psyllium (see p.156).

If you have fresh aloe vera growing in your garden, or know someone who does, you can make a potent intestinal and lower bowel cleanser by extracting the fresh juice. Simply cut a large leaf of aloe and scrape away the spiked edges, but do not peel. Cut into chunks, place in a blender, and purée. Squeeze the purée through a fine gauze cloth to extract the pure fluid, and discard the pulp. Take 1–2 tablespoons in a glass of water on an empty stomach, first thing in the morning and again at bedtime. If the purging effects are too strong, reduce the dosage; if not strong enough, increase it slightly. Fresh aloe juice may be used as a lower bowel cleansing supplement in conjuction with a detox diet, or taken occasionally as needed, for a week or two, to stimulate sluggish bowels, deal with chronic constipation or simply to give the colon a periodic purge.

During a detox programme, people with long-term bowel toxicity and other digestive disorders will sometimes experience an excess production of gas in the intestinal tract. This is caused by the activity of putrefactive bacteria as they are rousted from the bowels, by fermentation of dislodged toxic wastes, and by other biochemical reactions triggered in the digestive system by detox. If this becomes a problem, you may use herbs with 'carminative' properties to reduce gas reactions in the intestinal tract and relieve the flatulence it causes. A formula for carminative herbal tea to control gas is listed in Recipes and Formulas on page 334.

Lungs and bronchia: clearing the air vent

The lungs are known as the 'prime minister' of the internal organs, assisting the 'king' heart with the task of circulating blood through the body, and regulating pulse and blood pressure by virtue of diaphragmatic breathing. In addition to governing respiration and metabolism by supplying oxygen to the cells, the lungs also excrete carbon dioxide and other gaseous wastes from the body. The condition of the lungs is reflected externally in the skin: blemishes and other skin problems are often a manifestation of impaired lung function, and when both the lungs and the bowels are congested and clogged with mucus, toxic wastes are forced out of the body through the skin, causing further skin damage.

If a person has recently quit a long-term smoking habit, a detox programme will usually trigger a major expulsion of phlegm from the lungs and bronchia, as the body cleanses and repairs the lung tissues. This process may be assisted with the use of herbal expectorants, which help dissolve phlegm and propel it out of the lungs and bronchial tubes. 'Antitussive' herbs may be added to lung formulas to help control coughing and relieve sore throats, and 'demulcent' herbs can be included to soothe the inflammation of the mucous membranes which sometimes occurs as the lungs purge themselves of toxins, microbes and air pollutants.

Lungwort and pleurisy root are two of the most powerful herbs for decongesting and healing the lungs. Dragon River Herbals makes a very good herbal lung formula called Breath of Life, as a concentrated liquid extract, using lungwort, pleurisy root, osha root, horehound and other herbs with specific affinity for the lungs. In addition to detoxifying and decongesting the lungs and clearing the bronchial tubes, this formula also strengthens weak lungs, tones bronchial tissues and helps restore impaired lung functions.

In TCM, a tasty tea for clearing phlegm from the lungs may be prepared by boiling fresh ginger and dried liquorice root in water for 10 minutes, then straining out the liquid and adding a bit of honey to taste. This blend helps decongest the lungs and assists expectoration of phlegm from the bronchia. If persistent coughing is a problem during detox, you may use bee propolis in tincture form to soothe an itchy throat, control coughing and protect tender bronchial tissues from microbial infection. Simply stir ½ teaspoon of propolis tincture into 60–75 ml of hot water, add some honey to taste, and sip very slowly, so that it dribbles continuously down the throat.

One of the best forms of herbal therapy for detoxifying, decongesting and restoring the lungs and bronchial system during a detox programme is traditional Thai herbal steam, as discussed in Chapter 2 on page 60. All of the herbal steam blends given in the Recipes and Formulas section on page 324 help cleanse and clear the lungs, promote elimination of phlegm and pollutants from the bronchial tubes, and facilitate breathing and respiration.

If you don't have access to a herbal steamroom, you can improvise a steamer at home by placing a large pot of water on the stove, bringing it to the boil, then reducing the heat to a medium simmer. Add some aromatic herbs or essential oils with decongestant, bronchio-dilating properties, such as cinnamon, eucalyptus, peppermint, camphor and clove, then bend over the steaming pot holding a heavy bath towel like a tent over your head to trap the steam and enable you to inhale the aromatic vapours. This is an excellent way to clean the lungs and clear the bronchial passages on a daily basis during a detox programme; it can also be used any time in daily life to quickly decongest the lungs and open up the bronchia.

Brain and nerves: cleaning and balancing the circuits

Brain and nerve tissues are particularly susceptible to heavy metal and mineral toxicity. Owing to their electrical potential, brain and nerve cells attract heavy metals and other toxic metals like magnets. People who live and work either in densely populated urban areas or in highly industrialized regions, where factory and car exhaust pumps tons of toxic metals and minerals into the air every day, are very vulnerable to serious toxic damage to brain and nerve tissues from these sources. While virtually any type of detox diet or therapeutic fasting programme helps eliminate toxic metals and minerals from the brain and nerves, people who live in places that are heavily contaminated with these pollutants may wish to take extra measures to purge these poisons.

One of the best herbs for removing heavy metals from brain and nerve cells is coriander (cilantro), but it must be taken as a highly concentrated extract to be fully effective for this purpose. Coriander has a strong affinity for brain and nerve tissue, where it binds with and dislodges heavy metals clinging to neurons and nerve cells, allowing them to be flushed away in the blood and lymph. Dragon River Herbal produces a pure high-potency extract of coriander made specifically for this purpose; alternatively, you may ask someone who has the necessary skills and equipment to produce a concentrated coriander extract for you.

Ginkgo biloba has long been known for its powerful antioxidant activity in the brain and nervous system, for which it has specific natural affinity. Ginkgo may be taken as a tea, tablet or tincture to help clear the brain of toxic residues during a detox programme. It may also be used as a regular daily supplement to provide long-term antioxidant protection to the brain against damage from environmental toxins.

'Nervine' herbs, which calm the nervous system, promote sound sleep and restore balance to brain and nerve functions, can also be very helpful as supplemental support in a detox programme. During detox, the bloodstream must carry an overload of toxic substances from the tissues to the excretory organs, and as these toxins circulate through the system awaiting elimination, they can aggravate and overexcite the brain and nerves, causing nervous tension, irritability, insomnia and other symptoms of the 'detox blues'. When that occurs, the best solution is to take nervine herbal formulas that calm the nerves and soothe the brain, relax the mind and promote sound sleep. The body cannot remain in the state of rest and relaxation required to conduct detox and healing functions if the nervous system is 'jumpy' from excessive toxic exposure and the brain is buzzing with toxic tension. Nervine herbs can therefore play a pivotal role in a detox programme by preventing you from getting so wound up and impatient that you break your detox fast or cheat on your detox diet before completing it.

There are many excellent nervines in the herbal pharmacopoeia, including camomile, passion flower, catnip, hops, St John's wort, linden flowers, valerian and lavender. These may be taken singly or in various combinations as teas or tinctures, and some of them, such as lavender, may be used as essential oils for aromatherapy. A formula for nervine tea that may be taken daily to calm the nerves and keep body and mind relaxed during a therapeutic fast or in a detox diet program is provided in Recipes and Formulas on page 334. Several excellent nervine formulas in convenient liquid extract form are available from Dragon River Herbals, including a sound sleep formula called Lights Out and a relaxing nervine blend called Peace & Quiet.

Worms and parasites

Worms, intestinal flukes and dozens of other common parasites that enter and colonize the digestive tract generally don't cause much problem as long as they remain in the bowels and the internal 'climate' within the body remains properly balanced to keep them there. Serious problems can arise, however, when immune defences weaken and the tissues enter a state of chronic acidosis and hypoxia. When the body is highly toxic and resistance is low, worms and parasites flourish out of control and spread quickly to parts of the body where they are not supposed to go, such as the liver and brain.

All parasites feed and thrive on the body's own nutrients, robbing the human system of the essential nutrition it requires to sustain health, and excrete their toxic metabolic wastes into the body's tissues. Parasites are therefore a major source of blood and tissue toxicity, and as they multiply and spread, they gobble up an ever greater portion of the body's nutrients, further weakening the body's defences and polluting the internal terrain. Herbs which destroy worms and other parasites so that they may be eliminated from the system are known as 'anthelmintic', and they are very effective for ridding the body of these tenacious pests.

The most effective blend of herbs for overall worm and parasite control is the triplex formula of unripened black walnut hull, wormwood and clove. These herbs may be ground to a fine powder and taken in capsule form, or as concentrated liquid extracts, which are far more convenient. The triplex formula must be taken continuously for 2–3 months, in precise daily dosages, in order to achieve a complete eradication of all parasites, including the larva and eggs. When used in conjunction with the electronic 'Zapper' device introduced in the next chapter, the triplex formula effectively eradicates over a hundred varieties of parasite from every nook and cranny in the body. The Triplex tinctures are available in many herb shops and health stores, and may also be ordered by mail from Dragon River Herbals in the USA or Inner Glow Health Products in Australia. Be sure to ask your supplier to provide you with a copy of the proper dosage schedule.

Other herbs which help eliminate worms and parasites include pumpkin seed extract, gentian root, quassia bark, neem leaves, garlic and ginger. The latter two may be added fresh to all vegetable dishes during a detox diet to provide extra anthelmintic action; they may also be incorporated into your daily diet for ongoing protection against infestation by parasites.

'The people's medicine'

Traditional herbal medicine permits people to treat most of their own common health problems – including the root problem of tissue toxicity – safely and effectively at home, at far less cost and hazard to health than modern pharmaceutical drugs. In a study published by the World Health Organization (WHO) in 1992, medicinal herbs are described as 'the people's medicine'. The report states that 'medicinal plants offer . . . immediate access to safe and effective products for use in the treatment of illness by self-medication', and that 'the proper use of medicinal plants in therapy is a necessity, not a luxury.' As pathogens grow ever more resistant to the effects of chemical drugs, these drugs become less and less effective in controlling even the most superficial symptoms of disease, while also making the root problem of toxicity much worse – all at ever growing expense and risk to the consumer.

The reason that herbal medicine still remains 'the people's medicine' is because herbs cannot be patented, and therefore monopolized, by private pharmaceutical companies. Consequently, herbs remain affordable to almost everyone, and people can grow many of them in their own gardens at home. Moreover, some of the most effective medicinal herbs are also among the most common and inexpensive, and this is especially true of internal cleansing herbs. When body and mind remain relaxed and at rest and the nervous system switches over to the healing mode of the parasympathetic branch, the hormones, enzymes and other natural biochemicals produced in the body work in therapeutic synergy with the organic phytochemicals released into the system by medicinal herbs. As long as correct dietary and other guidelines are followed and medicinal herbs are properly selected and prepared, they always enhance the cleansing and healing process during detox, without causing the unpleasant and hazardous side effects invariably produced by chemical drugs.

Owing to their specific natural affinity for various organs and tissues in the body, medicinal herbs may be selected and blended with great precision to achieve particular therapeutic results in specifically targeted parts of the body. With a bit of common

sense and the aid of a good practical guide to the use of medicinal herbs at home, such as my book *A Handbook of Chinese Healing
Herbs* and Alma Hutchen's *A Handbook of Native American Herbs**,
almost anyone can formulate and prepare their own basic herbal
teas and boiled decoctions for detox purposes at home, or select
the right blends of herbal tablets and tinctures in any health
shop, exactly according to their own personal requirements.
While it's always best to also seek guidance from a qualified
health professional who specializes in herbal therapy, such guidance is not yet widely available in many parts of the world, so
those who wish to harness the healing power of herbs for detox
and healing at home must take 'the people's medicine' into their
own hands and administer it to their own bodies, along with
the other 'healing angels' of food, water, air and sunlight.

* Published by Shambhala Publications, Boston, USA; may be ordered
by mail through any bookshop or via the internet.

CHAPTER 9

High-Tech Electro-Detox

In addition to traditional methods of detoxifying and healing the human body, such as fasting, hydrotherapy, heliotherapy and herbs, there are now a variety of high-tech 'electro-detox' devices available, developed by independent medical researchers using the latest advances in modern electronics and computer technology. In fact, the alternative health care market has become flooded with new gadgets and gizmos that promise to cure you of everything from arthritis to Alzheimer's, and correct whatever else might be wrong with you as well, with the simple push of a button. Buyer beware! While traditional healing methods such as herbs and acupuncture are tried-and-tested therapies that have been proven safe and effective over time, many of these new electronic devices, with all their impressive bells and whistles and blinking lights, have no therapeutic value whatsoever, and some of them can even do you harm. It's always best, therefore, to exercise caution when selecting new high-tech tools for detox, and to consult with someone who has experience in their use. Properly applied, some of these electro-detox devices can greatly facilitate the cleansing and healing process, whilst also correcting basic imbalances in the human energy system that are the root cause of many physical disorders. As a result, it's well worth familiarizing yourself with some of these new technologies, and learning how to use them to assist the detox and healing process.

The human energy system

Since most electro-detox devices work through the human energy system, it's helpful to understand the basic principles of human energy. The entire human body and all its myriad parts operate on energy in much the same way that a complex mainframe computer runs on electricity. As long as all the circuits are open and sufficient power is running freely through the system, all the various functional sub-systems and moving parts operate smoothly. But as soon as there's a short-circuit somewhere in the energy network, or a blocked relay, blown fuse or rusted switch, the whole system goes 'haywire', and all sorts of strange symptoms begin to develop in the physical apparatus. It won't help to add some oil here, change a part there or fiddle with the dials: in order restore proper function, you must fix the root problem by finding and clearing the blockages in the energy system, rebalancing the circuits and restoring the power supply to all parts of the system.

The human energy system (HES) constitutes an invisible template of energy which powers and regulates the entire physical body. By using external sources of energy to recharge and rebalance the HES, each cell in every tissue of the body is revitalized and all vital functions are restored to normal. There are three basic dimensions to the HES. The one most directly related to organic functions of the body is the system of 12 organ-energy meridiens, which activate and control the vital organs and their related glands and tissues. This is the energy network used for acupuncture therapy in TCM. Another dimension of the HES is the chakra system, comprised of seven chakras, or 'energy wheels' stacked one above the other from coccyx to crown along the spinal column, like a pagoda of energy. Known as 'elixir

fields' (*dan-tien*) in TCM, the chakras function as energy transformers to 'step down' the ultra-high frequencies of cosmic
energy that radiate from sky to earth and enter the human system
through the crown chakra on top of the head. Each chakra
receives specific frequencies of these higher energies and transforms them into patterns and vibrational rates compatible with
the HES. They are then transmitted to energize specific functions
of both body and mind. Whenever a blockage or imbalance
develops in a particular chakra, the related physical and mental
functions become impaired, and the body grows vulnerable to
disease and degeneration.

The third aspect of human energy is known in TCM as *wei-chi*,
or 'guardian energy', which travels around the whole body just
below and above the surface of the skin, forming a protective
shield against invasive external energies. This surface shield of
guardian energy is the innermost core of the multi-layered
human energy field (HEF), which has numerous additional shells
of auric energy of increasingly subtler quality surrounding and
overlapping it. For the purposes of physical health and healing,
it's mainly this inner core of the HEF that's treated in bio-electric
energy medicine. With all the hazardous unnatural energies and
artifical electromagnetic fields in the environment today, the
protective role of guardian energy in fending off negative energies and resisting harmful force fields is more important than
ever to human health and longevity.

Internally, each and every one of the body's 75 trillion cells
functions like a micro-battery and has its own individual polarity
and energy field. Collectively, the sum total of all this cellular
energy determines the overall strength and radiance of guardian
energy field, and represents the net potential energy available
to the whole system. If a blockage or imbalance in the flow of
energy occurs in a particular part of the body due to damaged
or toxic tissues, trillions of cells are 'unplugged' from the energy
system and go 'off-line', deflating the guardian energy field and

drastically reducing the power supply to the whole system. This results in low immunity and weak resistance, and opens the gate to disease and invasive external energies.

The overall electrical potential of the HEF can easily be measured with an ordinary volt meter. A robust individual with the 'glow of good health' will register a significantly higher electrical potential than a weak and ailing individual, while a corpse doesn't even budge the meter's needle. Electromagnetic energy is one of the fundamental energies that activate the universe and everything in it. The HEF functions within the greater context of the earth's and the sun's electromagnetic fields, and is strongly influenced by any fluctuations in planetary and solar energies. The specific frequencies of electromagnetic energy that activate organic life are known to modern energy healers as 'bio-electric energy', or simply 'bio-energy'; in TCM it's called 'true energy'. It is this spectrum of bio-electric energy which electro-detox devices generate and transmit into the HES in order to recharge and rebalance it. The potential significance of these recent discoveries to the future of human health and healing is incalculable. As Dr Robert Becker, one of the world's leading authorities on human energy and bio-electric therapy, states:

> The data obtained in the past few years indicate very clearly that we must now include the Earth's normal geomagnetic field as an environmental variable of great consequence when we deal with the basic functions of living things . . . . It provides us with a key to the mechanisms by which all electromagnetic fields produce biological effects . . .

Dr Becker's research provides scientific confirmation of the ancient Chinese view of the human energy system as a complex network consisting of hundreds of energy channels and overlapping energy fields, which may be manipulated to transmit therapeutic energies into the human system to heal the body, balance the mind and correct deviations in the HES. Dr Becker has developed techniques to activate the body's innate self-cleansing and healing responses by applying electrical stimulation to the HEF, and he has invented electronic devices that may be used to accelerate the mending of broken bones and healing of traumatic wounds. These units produce precisely the correct wave patterns and energy frequencies required to signal the brain to activate and sustain internal cleansing and healing responses.

The hazards of 'energy pollution'

Just as toxic residues and acid wastes in the body pollute the blood and tissues, and negative thoughts and emotions disrupt the mind, so unnatural energies and harmful force fields in the environment 'pollute' the HES and tarnish the guardian energy field. Prior to the advent of modern industry and high-tech urban lifestyles, the only factors that disrupted the balance and integrity of the HES were the natural forces of 'heaven and earth', such as heat and cold, wind and rain, and sudden shifts in weather, as well as the pulses of the earth's electromagnetic field and cyclic fluctuations in solar radiation and other cosmic energies from the sky. Today, in addition to dealing with these natural forces, the HES must also defend itself against constant assault by far more aggressive and harmful forms of artificial 'energy pollution' produced by industry and modern technology. The entire environment today teems with invisible microwave radiation, unnatural radio frequencies, atomic radiation, artificial electromagnetic fields (EMF) produced by power lines and transformers, and other aberrant energies that cause severe deviations and imbalances in the HES. This sort of pollution is even more widespread and hazardous than ordinary air pollution because these toxic energies and unbalanced force fields penetrate glass and concrete and permeate all human habitats, outdoors as well as indoors. They also penetrate into the deepest tissues of the body. Today, there are 250 million times more artificially generated radio waves in the atmosphere than there were only 70 years ago, and microwave radiation from the mobile phone industry is polluting our energy environment to crisis proportions. Here's what Dr Robert Becker has to say about microwaves:

> The scientific data at this time indicate that microwaves have major biological effects at power levels *far below* those required to cause heating [such as as those used in microwave ovens]. The majority of these effects are productive of various disease states, primarily cancer and genetic defects. . . . The hazard comes from the fact that exposure to microwaves, like exposure to any abnormal electromagnetic field, produces stress, a decline in immune system competency, and changes in the genetic apparatus. Thus, the levels of exposure that the government says are 'safe' are in fact not safe at all.

Think about that the next time you make a call on your mobile or heat something up in a microwave oven.

High-voltage power lines, which operate at 60 hertz, create an artificial EMF of 100 milligauss that extends 20 metres in every direction around them. The level of exposure to artificial EMF above which cancer and brain damage can occur has been determined to be 3 milligauss. Writes Dr Becker, 'At this time, the scientific evidence is absolutely conclusive: 60 hertz magnetic fields cause human cancer cells to permanently increase their rate of growth by as much as 1,600 per cent and to develop more malignant characteristics.'

Common household appliances such as televisions, computers, hair dryers, electric shavers and the like further contaminate the human energy environment with artificial EMF ranging up to 100 milligauss in strength. A good example of the sort of health hazard this poses is the fact that women who work as professional beauticians and hairdressers are known to suffer an unusually high rate of breast cancer, and a major causative factor is the electric hair dryer they hold only centimetres from their breasts for hours each day. One shudders to think what damage this does to their customer's brain cells, as at a distance of 15 cm a typical electric hair dryer generates a blazing artificial EMF of 50 milligauss.

The net result of chronic exposure to these various forms of invisible artificial energy pollution is an ongoing onslaught against the balance and strength of the HES and its surrounding bio-field, and a constant challenge to health that drains the whole system of vitality. These abnormal fields and energy frequencies disrupt vital functions, weaken immune response, disturb the mind and drive the whole human system further into a state of energy imbalance that contributes much to blood acidosis and tissue toxicity. Traditional energy medicine such as acupuncture, heliotherapy, aromatherapy and breathing, which utilize natural energies to deal with natural imbalances in the human system, are often insufficient to deal with the deeper deviations in the HES caused by artificial EMF, intensive microwave radiation and other sources of unnatural energy pollution. When the HES has been damaged and the bio-field deranged by chronic exposure to these hazardous artificial energies, often the best recourse is to 'fight fire with fire' by applying the latest advances in high-tech electro-detox therapies.

Prescription for 'Bio-electric energy medicine'

The primacy of energy over matter as the most decisive factor in human health and life in general has been proven beyond doubt in scientific theory and clinical practice, but the mainstream medical industry still clings stubbornly to its vested interests in the chemical/mechanical approach of allopathic and surgical medicine, and continues to turn a blind eye to these new discoveries. But that has not prevented the inventive wizards of high-tech alternative medical science from forging ahead on their own to develop new healing technologies based on the view of the human body as a dynamic, interactive bioelectric energy field, and to devise devices that allow prescriptions for bio-electric energy medicine to be delivered safely into the human energy system.

The tricky part of this new bio-electric medical technology is to accurately replicate the precise frequencies, currents and wave patterns of human energy, to reproduce their intricate pulses and complex rhythms, and to introduce these externally generated energies into the human bio-field. While many of the new gadgets on the market today are useless, and sometimes even hazardous, there are several recently developed devices that have demonstrated remarkable results as therapeutic tools for detoxifying, repairing and rebalancing the human body.

In previous chapters, we briefly discussed how two of these new inventions – the GEOMED Activated Air System, and the alkalized, ionized micro-clustered water system – use electric energy to boost the potency of air and water as cleansing and healing elements in the body. In the following pages, we'll take a look at five more high-tech electro-detox devices that may be safely and effectively used in conjunction with traditional therapies to enhance and hasten cleansing and healing functions during a detox programme. These methods have all been extensively tested and proven therapeutically effective in clinical practice, and they may also be safely used at home.

The Jai electro-pressure
regeneration therapy

The Jai device is a small, pocket-sized, battery-operated unit which produces a gentle wave of electrons that sweeps through the body's tissues and recharges each and every cell with 'electro-pressure'. Driven by currents that are compatible with the natural bio-electric energies of the HES, the Jai delivers detoxifying antioxidant activity to the whole system and stimulates rapid healing of wounds and damaged organs. Clinical studies have shown that the Jai unit accelerates the rate of healing in elderly people and brings it up to par with that of youth by regenerating the body's ability to cleanse and repair itself.

As previously noted, water has a unique capacity to record and transmit any energy patterns and frequencies to which it is exposed. The Jai takes advantage of the natural conductivity of water by using it as a medium in which an externally generated electric charge interacts with the bio-electric charge of the human energy field in order to produce therapeutic effects in the human system. Acting as a sympathetic mediator between the body's energy field and the healing field produced by the Jai device, the water generates a bio-electric energy field which harmonizes the HEF with the incoming energy waves from the unit, thereby creating a therapeutically beneficial bio-electric field. This is achieved by soaking absorbent foam-padded bands in water, wrapping them snugly around the wrists or ankles, where the patterns and pulses of the HES broadcast most clearly, then attaching an electrode from the unit to each band. This allows the incoming electric charge to interact and blend with the patterns of the HES imprinted in the water within the bands. Adapting the external charge to the precise conditions of human energy, the water conducts the signals from the resulting balanced bio-field directly into the body, where they enter the energy channels, which in turn deliver the precisely programmed therapeutic energy pulses to the whole system.

Electro-pressure regeneration therapy provides manifold benefits to human health and longevity. The incoming bio-electric charge opens the energy meridiens, increases energy flow and balances energy distribution throughout the system. It relieves pain and reduces inflammation in the soft tissues of the body, promotes rapid healing of wounds and elevates immune response. The Jai's potent antioxidant activity mops up free radicals and neutralizes toxins throughout the body, which makes it particularly effective as a supporting therapy for any type of detox programme. Unlike nutritional and herbal antioxidants, which depend on the vagaries of the digestive and circulatory systems for delivery, electro-pressure regeneration therapy overrides the physical pathways and delivers its vigorous anti-oxidant activity directly to every tissue and cell of the body via the bio-electric template of the HES. The Jai may also be used in the course of daily life for a quick, convenient mini-detox, and to recharge and rebalance the whole system whenever energy runs low.

The BEFE bio-electric bath

Q-Tech of Australia has recently developed an electromagnetic device that programmes ordinary water as a powerful tool for detoxification and healing. This system, known as the Bio-Electric Field Enhancer (BEFE), utilizes bathwater as a medium to cleanse the lymphatic system and rebalance the entire human energy field. In TCM, the 'true energy' that activates the human body is regarded as the essential force of life, the fundamental foundation of health and the primary key to healing. This is the energy that the BEFE unit manipulates in order to stimulate detox and healing responses in the human body.

Like the Jai device, BEFE technology utilizes water as a medium to transfer healing energy signals into the body and rebalance the human energy field. Since water reproduces and holds the precise patterns and vibratory rates of any energy field to which it's exposed, when the human body – which itself is over 70 per cent water – is submerged in a tub of water, the body's bio-energy field imprints itself and produces an exact personal 'energy profile' in the water, including all the imbalances and deviations that require correcting. At the same time, the BEFE unit introduces a perfectly balanced, properly tuned bio-energy field into the water, where it interfaces and interacts with the body's energy field, correcting imbalances and adjusting abnormalities in the latter until the two fields harmonize and resonate as one in the water. When the body's bio-energy field has been recharged and rebalanced by the externally generated bio-electric field in the water, the physical body responds immediately to the properly balanced signals by detoxifying and repairing itself. Note that BEFE therapy may be applied in a foot bath as well, with equally effective results.

By correcting faulty circuits in the HES and restoring balance in the body's bio-field, BEFE therapy triggers a major cleansing response through the skin, drawing toxic residues and acid wastes out from the subcuteneous tissues and lymph channels, and excreting them through the skin into the bathwater. Naturopathic healers in Australia who have used this device in their clinical practice report that after only 20–30 minutes of therapy some of their more toxic clients turn the bathwater brown with toxic wastes excreted through the skin. This is powerful detox technology, and it's best to seek some professional guidance when using it at home, or else to try it at a naturopathic clinic or spa first.

The Zapper

In the course of her research into the hazards posed to human health from infestation by common parasites, particularly the nasty fluke (*Fasciolopsis buskii*), which uses the human intestinal tract as a breeding and picnic ground, Dr Hulda Clarke has developed a small, battery-operated device which generates an 8-volt current of 30 Khz with a square wave pattern, precisely tuned to destroy, or 'zap', these tenacious parasites, without harming the human body. This Neuro Muscle Stimulator, popularly known as the Zapper, may be used in conjunction with the Triplex herbal parasite formula introduced in the previous chapter, for even better results.

According to Dr Clarke and many other naturopathic healers, one of the primary causes of some of the world's most virulent and often fatal ailments is the extreme tissue toxicity produced by the poisonous secretions and metabolic wastes which flukes and other parasites release inside the body. Common debilitating conditions such as asthma, cancer, chronic fatigue syndrome and candida fungal infections often develop as a direct result of parasite infestation, and whenever parasites are the primary cause of these ailments, the only effective cure is a complete eradication of all parasites in the body. This is the purpose for which the Zapper was invented. Victims of chronic asthma and candida infection usually respond quickly to anti-parasite therapy, and several lifelong asthmatics in Australia who used the Zapper for this purpose reported that they no longer needed to use inhalers and could breathe freely again after only ten weeks' treatment.

When using the Zapper, it's important to follow carefully the treatment protocol. Treatments are usually done in three consecutive sessions of 7 minutes each, with a 15-minute pause in between. The reason for this sequence is that some of the parasites inside the human body carry smaller parasites within themselves, and when they're 'zapped' and killed by the incoming electric wave, they release these other parasites directly into the body, some of which are even more toxic to human tissues than their hosts. The second round of treatment is therefore needed to knock out these hidden fellow travellers, and the third round to mop up any survivors of the first two rounds. Dr Clarke's recommended treatment schedule for a complete elimination of parasites is as follows:

> **Week 1:**   One session per day of three consecutive 7-minute periods, with a 15-minute pause in between.
>
> **Week 2:**   One session per day of only one 7-minute period.
>
> **Week 3:**   One session every two days of only one 7-minute period, for a total of 3 times in the week.
>
> **Week 4:**   One session per week of only one 7-minute period, in conjunction with the commencement of the Triplex herbal formula.

For even better results, this programme may be done while following a strict detox diet to accelerate elimination of the dead parasites and all the metabolic waste they leave in the blood and tissues. Once a complete eradication of parasites has been achieved, a series of treatments of one to three weeks duration every six to 12 months usually suffices to keep the body free of parasites, especially if the daily diet is reformed to eliminate the internal conditions of acidosis and toxaemia in which parasites thrive. Other maintenance protocols with the Zapper include one session once a week, or three consecutive days of one session each every month. While the Zapper is very effective used alone, when combined with the Triplex herbal formula, it eliminates a wider range of parasites and penetrates more deeply into the tissues.

The Zapper should not be used by people with pacemakers or other electronic implants, nor by pregnant women. Other than that, it is safe to use at any time by people who wish to rid their bodies of parasites and eliminate the diseases and degenerative conditions they cause. There are several models on the market and a variety of treatment protocols, so be sure to get one that has been properly manufactured and tested for quality control, and always follow the directions provided with the unit.

The NET: no more 'cold turkey'

One of the most important new inventions in the field of electro-energy medicine, particularly in terms of its potential applications for dealing with a major worldwide health crisis is neuro-electric therapy, or NET. It's also a perfect example of how the 'best of East and West' may be successfully blended in medical therapy, and how fusing the ancient healing principles of Asia with the modern technology of the West can achieve greater therapeutic results than either one could ever produce alone.

The NET technology was inspired by a fortunate stroke of serendipity. The Scottish surgeon Dr Margaret 'Meg' Patterson was working at a hospital in Hong Kong during the late 1970s, where she observed Western-trained Chinese surgeons using electrically enhanced acupucture to help their patients recover more swiftly and less painfully in post-surgery. She also observed that some of these patients persistently pestered their doctors to keep them hooked onto the electro-acupuncture unit all the time, day and night, and that without it they became extremely restless and irritable. Later, a few of them finally admitted that they were in fact long-term heroin or opium addicts whose habits had been abruptly interrupted by their surgery, forcing them to endure acute drug withdrawal symptoms that were all the more agonizing after the trauma of surgery. They explained that whenever the electro-acupuncture therapy was applied, the 'cold turkey' of withdrawal symptoms vanished within minutes.

Subsequently, Dr Patterson went to America and approached Dr Robert Becker to research this phenomenon. Before long, they discovered that the key factor which produced the immediate relief from withdrawal symptoms was neither the acupuncture needles nor the points needled, but rather the pulsing electric current which the needles transmitted into the body. Soon afterwards Dr Patterson developed the NET device, which is about the same size as the Jai unit and attaches to the body with two small electrodes patched to the mastoid bone behind each ear. The NET device generates a gentle micro-current of precisely the same frequencies and wave patterns produced by the brain when under the influence of a particular addictive drug. The genius of Dr Patterson's work lies in the fact that she managed to precisely map the exact energy frequencies and brain wave patterns associated with each addictive drug – heroin, cocaine, amphetamines, barbiturates and alcohol – then produced a small computer chip for each one, which pre-programmes the NET device for the specific drug addiction to be treated.

After the addict takes his or her last dose of the drug and is ready for detox and withdrawal, the NET is patched to the body and remains attached day and night, except for showers, for the full ten days required to effect complete withdrawal. During this time, it delivers a continuous current of soothing neuro-electric therapy to the brain. The frequencies and wave patterns produced by the NET prevent the patient from experiencing the worst symptoms of drug withdrawal, and at the same time enable the body to remain completely drug-free throughout the course of treatment, allowing it to swiftly and effectively detoxify itself. By the time the treatment is terminated ten days later, the body has already passed painlessly beyond the most critical stage of drug withdrawal, without the intolerable trauma of 'cold turkey', and without the need to use substitute drugs such as methadon or sedatives, which not only re-enforce addictive behaviour but also prevent the detox process taking place.

Despite a consistent cure rate of over 90 per cent in frequently repeated clinical trials, the medical establishments in America and most other Western nations still refuse to approve it for official drug withdrawal programmes. Because NET therapy requires no expensive drugs, no clinical treatment and no dependence on doctors – i.e. because it works so well – it poses a major threat to many powerful vested interests in the medical industry, and so far only Ireland, Germany and one or two other countries have officially certified its use.

The NET definitely works, as Rolling Stones guitarist Keith Richards, singer Boy George and numerous other rock celebrities who were once stubbornly addicted to heroin can attest. Dr Meg, as she's affectionately known to those she's helped, has gifted the world the most effective drug detox method ever developed. However, until government health agencies and medical establishments acknowledge the proven efficacy of NET therapy, and sanction its clinical use for drug and alcohol withdrawal programmes, those who wish to use this method must seek treatment through private channels.

Radionics: re-balancing the body's bio-electric field

Radionics is a new energy medicine technology that works with the specific spectrums of universal energy associated with the human system. Radionics therapy is based on the scientifically proven principles that everything in the universe, from atoms to stars and microbes to humans, ultimately boils down to the same fundamental component – energy – and that each particular form of energy is governed by its own unique intrinsic data field (IDF), which determines its characteristcs and regulates its activity. Dr Karl Jacobs, an energy healer who specializes in radionics therapies at his Villa Deva energy medicine clinic in Chiang Mai, Thailand, explains it as follows:

The references to this spectrum have been given many names, such as radionics, psionics, dowsing, bioplasm, bio-electric energy, bio-fields and Intrinsic Data Fields, as well as *chi* and *prana* in traditional Asian medicine. Regardless of the name, these subtle energy fields, or 'bio-fields', are said to contain the essential 'intelligence', or information, which provides the distinctive pattern, or 'energy matrix', that determines the organization of a particular form of matter. We call these informational patterns 'Intrinsic Energy Fields', and in many instances they explain phenomena that cannot be explained by conventional medical science.

The device most commonly used to apply radionics therapy is called the SE-5, which is a compact, computer-based electronic instrument about the size of a laptop computer. This device, also known as a bio-field analyser, is programmed to detect and correct imbalances in the HEF and clear negative energies from the HES, thereby eliminating the root cause of many physical, mental and emotional disorders and restoring optimum energy balance to the whole human system.

The SE-5 may also be used to increase the therapeutic potency of essential oils and herbal extracts to produce therapeutically energized 'elixirs', to programme crystals with specific healing energy frequencies, and to clear negative energies from homes, offices and other human habitats. Generally, the radionics therapist will ask the client to provide a lock of hair or a fingernail clipping, which is used to 'tune in' the SE-5's sensors to the unique identifying frequencies of the client's personal energy system. 'Radionics is a powerful tool for healing,' states Dr Jacobs. 'When you sign up for a consultation or a private cleansing retreat with me, I will ask for a sample of your hair, and from this I will determine which elixirs to create specifically for you, and prepare a comprehensive programme of personal priorities designed to help you achieve your optimum state of health and well-being.'

Since radionics therapy operates entirely in the dimension of energetics, consultations may be done long-distance, simply by mailing a hair sample to the therapist, who then analyzes the client's bio-energy field, prepares the precise energized elixirs required to correct imbalances and clear blockages in the client's energy system, and mails them back to the client. Anyone interested in further information about radionics, or in arranging a consultation, may visit Dr Jacobs' website: www.cleanse4life.com

'New wave, same sea'

High-tech energy medicine is certainly a 'new wave' of the future in human healing and preventive health care, and it's particularly effective for repairing damage and correcting deviations in the HES caused by high-tech energy pollution, such as artificial EMF, microwaves and unnatural radio frequencies. Nevertheless, it's important to remember that regardless of how sophisticated and 'advanced' these high-tech devices become, the therapeutic energies they generate still come from the same 'sea' of basic universal energy of which the human body has always been composed and of which traditional holistic medicine has been aware for thousands of years.

Rarely does high-tech electro-detox therapy by itself suffice to achieve effective and lasting results in healing the human system. In order for these new bio-electric energy technologies to achieve optimum results and effect permanent cures, they must always be applied in close conjunction with diet and nutrition, breathing and exercise, water and sunlight, and other traditional therapies that work directly with the fundamental energies and elements of the human system. High-tech electro-detox, and bio-electric energy medicine in general, are still in their infancy, and so far only a few of these new technologies have established a proven track record of therapeutic efficacy. The devices introduced above are among those that have demonstrated the most consistent positive results in clinical use as well as at home.

In fact, in some cases, these new technologies can make the crucial difference between success and failure in a detox and healing programme. Neuro-electric therapy (NET), for example, has repeatedly proven itself to be the key factor in curing the most stubborn cases of drug and alcohol addiction, because it permits detox to proceed without trauma and without resort to other drugs. The Zapper can be a decisive factor in curing conditions caused by long-term parasite infestation, and the GEOMED Activated Air System promises to become an indispensable tool for treating respiratory and other ailments that arise from chronic deficiency in the essential energy of negative ions in the air, especially in polluted cities. Still, when choosing detox and healing therapies, it's always best to begin with the most basic elements of life in the body, such as food, herbs, water, air and sunlight, then amplify and accelerate those therapies with synergistic high-tech electro-detox methods.

PART 2

'Retox'

CHAPTER 10

The Art of Rational Retox

Let's face it: life on earth is toxic. No sooner is detox done than retox resumes. The moment you start eating normally again, your digestive system starts producing toxic wastes, cellular metabolism re-pollutes the bloodstream with carbon dioxide and acid residues, exercise sours the muscles with lactic acid and the whole process of progressive tissue toxicity begins once more.

The body's internal self-cleansing mechanisms are designed to deal with these natural sources of tissue toxicity on a daily basis through normal excretory functions, but it's not equipped to handle the heavy overload of inorganic toxins and putrefactive wastes produced by unnatural sources of internal pollution such as chemically processed foods and medicines, toxic air and water, and indigestible combinations of denatured foods. For most people today, tissue toxicity is further aggravated by relentless enervation of the nervous system from chronic stress, insufficient rest and relaxation, overstimulation of the senses and excessive dependence on stimulants and intoxicants. These stress factors keep the autonomic nervous system constantly racing in the 'fight or flight' sympathetic mode, exhausting the adrenal glands, weakening immune response and flooding the bloodstream with highly acid-forming residues from stress hormones and the toxic metabolites they produce in the tissues.

Unable to process and eliminate this growing overload of toxins through 'normal channels', the body is instead forced to store them in joints and bones, liver and bowels, fat and lymph, and any other tissue where they cannot directly poison the blood-stream. If these toxic deposits are not periodically dislodged from the tissues in which they're stored and flushed out of the body, it's only a matter of time before they do serious damage to those tissues and cause cellular malfunctions that can lead to cancer, heart disease, Alzheimer's disease, and other fatal conditions.

The only viable solution to the modern problem of toxicity in daily life is to cultivate the 'art of rational retox'. In a nutshell, this means redesigning your lifestyle so that it minimizes internal pollution and maximizes internal cleansing functions. It means reforming your daily diet and re-ordering your daily priorities. In order to do this, you must take the time to learn how your body works, paying close attention to how it reacts to the various things you feed it and do to it. You need to consider the 'cost/benefit' factors involved in what you eat, drink and do each day, and learn to avoid those things whose cumulative costs to health and longevity far outweigh their benefits. Practising the art of 'rational retox' in your daily life can make the crucial difference between long-term health and longevity and chronic disease and degeneration, especially when practised in conjunction with periodic detox diets or therapeutic fasts.

The great advantage in doing a detox programme first, prior to trying to eliminate harmful food addictions and reform bad eating habits, is that a preliminary detox makes it much easier to break unhealthy food addictions and cultivate healthy new eating habits. People who suddenly stop eating sugar, meat or dairy products without first purging their bowels, blood and tissues of the toxic residues left by these foods in the body usually find it difficult to resist the craving for these things, and almost impossible to stick strictly to their new diets. That's because physiologically food addictions are very similar to drug addictions. The body grows accustomed to their metabolic effects and learns to tolerate the damage they do. In some cases, such as sugar addiction, the nervous system becomes dependent on the toxic by-products of sugar metabolism, which act as nervous stimulants. When these substances are abruptly withdrawn from the body, their toxic residues remain in the blood and tissues, leaving a 'metabolic memory' that intoxicates the mind with cravings for them. While the symptoms of withdrawal from food addictions are not as intense and dramatic as those produced by drugs, they are nevertheless very similar, and include hypertension, insomnia, headaches, indigestion, depression and irritability. By doing a detox programme to purify the blood and tissues and completely rid the body of all toxic 'leftovers' from former food habits, all withdrawal symptoms are eliminated in a single week of detox, during which time you have nothing else to do anyway but pamper yourself with hot saltwater baths, herbal steams, deep-tissue massages and other soothing detox protocols to ease the cleansing symptoms. By the time the detox programme is done, all cravings for former dietary habits and food addictions will have totally disappeared, and healthy new eating habits and food choices may be cultivated to replace them.

If you find it difficult to give up all unhealthy eating habits and harmful food choices after your first round of detox, then just try eliminating one or two, and work on the others later, after your next detox programme. As the novelist Nelson Algren observed, 'Life is hard by the yard, but a cinch by the inch'. This is especially true when it comes to replacing old ways with new. But if you take it step by step, replacing wrong choices with right ones, one by one, you will soon discover that good habits are as easy to cultivate as bad ones, and just as hard to break, and that a healthy diet and wholesome lifestyle can be even more habit-forming than indiscriminate self-indulgence.

Detox/retox

The first step in the art of rational retox is to re-design your diet and other daily lifestyle factors in ways that allow your body to unload most of its toxic wastes on a daily basis, rather than letting them accumulate inside and cause blood acidosis and tissue toxicity. The more efficiently the body detoxifies itself daily, the fewer toxins remain stored in the tissues, and the easier each periodic detox programme becomes. To put it another way, the more you let your body heal itself daily, the less severe is the 'healing crisis' later when you do an intensive cleansing programme. Efficient daily detox also makes life a lot more pleasant and productive by increasing available energy, boosting physical vitality and enhancing mental clarity.

Although retox is a natural process of life that functions automatically, you can take rational measures to slow down the rate of retoxification and lessen the impact of internal pollution. In addition, the extent to which you practise such preventive measures can have a decisive influence on overall health and longevity. Detox is also a natural function of the body, but it's only designed to process toxic wastes from natural sources. In order to deal with the heavy overload of unnatural toxins that today collect in the human body from pollutants in food, water, air, medicines and other environmental sources, you must take extra steps to help your body to eliminate these poisons on a daily basis, thereby protecting yourself from the damage they produce if they are allowed to accumulate inside. These toxic chemical residues from industrial sources pollute the bloodstream and corrode the tissues far more swifty and severely than natural metabolic wastes, and failure to periodically flush them from the body paves a quick path to disease, degeneration and premature death.

The key elements required to produce precisely the right 'climate' within the body for detox and self-cleansing mechanisms to operate continuously day and night are alkali and oxygen. As long as the blood and tissues remain sufficiently alkalized and oxygenated, they will naturally cleanse and rebalance themselves, and the body will be able to neutralize and eliminate toxins as soon as they appear. Among the measures that may be taken to keep the blood and tissues alkalized and oxygenated on a daily basis, by far the most effective is proper utilization of life's two most basic elements – air and water – which flow through the body constantly, day and night. Correctly used, air and water continuously alkalize and oxygenate the body as they enter the system, and continuously eliminate toxic residues and acid wastes on the way out.

To facilitate daily detox in today's modern world, nothing works faster and more efficiently than drinking the alkalized, ionized, micro-clustered water (microwater) introduced in Chapter 2 (see page 43). Drinking this type of activated water throughout the day and using it to prepare all your foods and beverages provides continuous internal detox and cleansing activity that permeates all the tissues and fluids of the body, and allows the cells to eliminate their metabolic wastes as soon as they're produced. The negative charge carried by ionized water neutralizes toxic residues in the blood and tissues owing to its potent antioxidant properties, and the micro-clustered minerals and water molecules easily penetrate cellular membranes to keep all of the tissues sufficiently hydrated and mineralized and enable the body to maintain proper pH balance in the cellular fluids.

Negative ions also constitute the essential element in air which helps keep the body alkaline and oxygenated and facilitates continuous internal detox. When the oxygen molecules in the air we breathe are ionized, they become far more bio-active in the body, and their cleansing and healing properties become much stronger. The negative ion count in air is an accurate measure of its capacity to support life, and without that energy air is just a cocktail of inert gases. Breathing 'dead air' with low or no negative ion count is a major contributing factor to chronic fatigue, chronic toxaemia and chronic degeneration of the body, and as a result it's become one of the biggest hazards to human health today. Living in a forest high in the mountains, or on an unspoiled beach by the open sea, is no doubt the best solution to the problem, but it's simply not possible for most people to do that. The next best solutions, which are ones any of us can opt for, are to recharge dead air in homes and offices using negative ion generators, or to spend 30–60 minutes each day breathing purified, super-charged air from the GEOMED Activated Air System.

In addition to breathing bio-active air, it's also very important to learn how to breathe correctly, by using the diaphragm to draw the breath deep down into the abdomen, rather than breathing only in the narrow part of the upper chest. Correct diaphragmatic breathing greatly increases oxygenation of the blood and tissues, as well as elimination of carbon dioxide. It also has an immediate alkalizing effect on the bloodstream, thereby counteracting acidosis and assisting detox with each and every breath.

Besides air and water, other factors of daily life, such as food and supplements, may also be used to help keep the blood and tissues alkaline and assist the body's self-cleansing functions. Freshly extracted raw vegetable juices are particularly fast and effective alkalizers; including a glass or two each day in your diet is a very good way to prevent acidosis and facilitate rapid elimination of toxic wastes. Various dietary supplements may also be used as sources of elements that alkalize and detoxify blood and tissues, including all green foods such as chlorella, spirulina and cereal grass juices, also Celtic sea salt and marine mineral extracts, and antioxidant nutrients such as vitamins C and E, betacarotene, zinc and selenium. Sunlight, too, plays a vital role in this process by stimulating the body to produce enough vitamin D to ensure maximum assimilation of calcium from food, water and mineral supplements. Since calcium is the body's primary internal alkalizing agent and an essential element in all detox processes, sunlight can be an important supporting factor in maintaining the body's daily defence mechanisms against acidosis and toxaemia.

When all is said and done, however, it is usually diet that is the primary factor in the complex equations of detox/retox that determine human health. 'You are what you eat' is more than just a slick slogan: it's a basic fact of life. Rebalancing your diet according to the principles of trophology – the science of food combining – and reviewing your food choices in light of the effects they have on pH balance and other vital conditions in the body are the first and second steps on the path of rational retox. The reason that diet is the chief priority is simple: wrong food combinations and wrong food choices have become the primary causes of blood acidosis and tissue toxaemia, and these in turn are the primary conditions for the onset of disease and degeneration of the body. Once unhealthy food addictions have been given up, and acid-forming eating habits have been broken, cultivating healthy new eating habits becomes enjoyable and it is easy to develop a taste for wholesome alkalizing foods that nourish and balance the body rather than derange and ruin it.

In the following chapter, we'll review the most important rules for combining food in ways that minimize internal toxicity and maximize digestive efficiency. We'll then examine the major categories of food in light of both their effects and side effects within the body, and decide what's really healthy and safe to eat today and what's not.

CHAPTER 11

Food: Retox Diet and Supplements

Diet and nutrition are the primary building blocks in the foundation of human health and longevity, and the essential elements of life provided by food cannot be replicated or replaced with any form of modern technology. Owing to mass production and corporate control of the world's food supplies over the past century, the human diet has become as polluted with toxic wastes as everything else produced by the modern consumer industry. The industrially refined foods that most people consume today are contaminated with poisonous pesticides and preservatives, chemically altered with artificial flavours and colouring agents, and further denatured by irradiation and genetic modification. In the refinement process, most of the essential nutrients are stripped from the food, and the few that remain have little or no nutritional value. Prior to the advent of chemically processed foods, the famous American physician Dr Charles Mayo, founder of the Mayo Clinic, described the central role of wholesome food in human health as follows:

> Normal resistance to disease is directly dependent upon adequate food, normal resistance to disease never comes out of pill boxes. Adequate food is the cradle of normal resistance, the playground of normal

immunity, the workshop of good health, and the laboratory of long life.

Modern Western eating habits, particularly the fast-food and snack-diet approach propagated by the American food industry, are far from 'adequate' sources of nutrition for human health. These diets are composed almost entirely of the three most acid-forming types of food: animal products (meat, fat, eggs and dairy products); refined white starch (white bread, pastries, potatoes and starchy snack foods); and refined white sugar (sweets, ice cream, cakes, biscuits and sugary soft drinks). In North America, Western Europe and Australia, these three categories of food account for over 90 per cent of the calories consumed by most people; they also contribute to at least 90 per cent of the diseases and degenerative conditions people in those countries suffer. Overwhelmingly imbalanced in favour of highly acid-forming foods such as meat, milk, sugar and starch, and virtually devoid of the alkalizing elements found in fresh fruit and vegetables, modern Western diets saturate the human body with toxic acid wastes, poison the blood and tissues, weaken resistance and immunity and fling open the gates to chronic disease and degenerative conditions. The only way to deal with this daily dietary threat to health and longevity is to rationally re-design your diet and reform your eating habits in ways that reduce formation of acid wastes and increase alkalinity. This means re-ordering your priorities in food choices and adopting the basic laws of food combining to govern your eating habits.

The yin and the yang of it

The science of combining food in ways that prevent acid-forming reactions of fermentation and putrefaction in the digestive tract, while increasing alkalinity and reducing production of toxic wastes, is known in nutritional science as trophology. Following these principles in your daily diet and personal eating habits is the first basic step in applying the 'art of rational retox' to your daily life. Proper food combining is one of the most effective measures one can take to prevent the development of blood acidosis and tissue toxaemia, and it provides a practical way to control the balance of acid and alkaline elements in the body.

In TCM, the 'great principle of yin and yang', which lies at the heart of all functions of life, manifests its polar dynamics in diet and digestion in the form of alkaline (yin) and acid (yang) balance. As we can see from this terminology, traditional Chinese physicians regarded 'alkaline' as a manifestation of the cooling, calming, nourishing 'water' element of yin, and 'acid' as a reflection of the heating, agitating, depleting 'fire' element of yang. From this viewpoint, modern Western diets are extremely imbalanced with an excess of highly acid-forming yang foods such as meat, milk, eggs, fat, sugar and starch. This imbalance is further aggravated by the acidifying effects of eating these foods in wrong combinations, which drives the internal organs ever deeper into the inferno of what TCM calls 'fire-energy excess' (*huo-chi da*). The obvious solution to this problem of excess acid-forming yang is to rebalance the diet in the direction of more alkaline-forming yin factors.

Strictly applied, trophology becomes a highly complex discipline that can interfere with the enjoyment of food. Since everything we eat reacts in either a yin or yang way with anything else we eat together with it, as well as with whatever is already in the stomach, we can reach the point, if we're too fastidious about food combining, where we dare to eat only one single type of food at a time. This is impractical as well as boring, and it detracts from the natural pleasure of eating. Fortunately, it's also unnecessary. It's possible to compose meals that are properly balanced trophologically, as well as fully satisfying gastronomically, by following the '75 per cent rule', whereby the basic laws of food combining govern about 75 per cent of your food choices whenever you compose a meal, allowing you a 25 per cent margin of error for indiscriminate self-indulgence. This is a rational approach to food combining that is both practical and effective, and it may be applied with equal ease at home or in a restaurant.

For example, if the rule states, 'Don't combine meat and starch at the same meal', you don't need to be fanatical about it, plucking out the few slivers of chicken or prawns you find in a Chinese stir-fried dish that's over 90 per cent noodles and vegetables. Nor need you worry about having just one small wholegrain roll with a meal of meat and lots of vegetables. On the other hand, eating a large baked potato slathered with soured cream together with a thick steak or a greasy cheeseburger on a starchy white bun, is definitely a violation of the rules, punishable by acid indigestion and other gastric distress.

To simplify matters for those of you who wish to try trophology as a way of preventing indigestion, controlling internal acidity and reducing tissue toxicity, the most important rules for balancing alkaline-forming yin and acid-forming yang in diet on the basis of proper food combining are presented below in terms of their practical applications to six major categories of food: complex animal proteins, starchy carbohydrates, fats, sugars, fruits and vegetables.

Putrefactive protein

What we're discussing here is the complex, concentrated protein found in foods from animal sources, such as meat, fish and fowl, eggs and dairy products, not the light, simple protein contained in nuts and seeds, beans and grains, and other vegetable sources. Vegetable proteins are far less complex and condensed than animal protein, and are therefore much easier to digest. They also combine well with most other foods. Meat, eggs and dairy products, on the other hand, cause digestive disaster when wrongly combined with other foods, or even when improperly combined with each other.

The first and foremost rule of food combining is: 'Don't eat concentrated animal protein and starchy carbohydrates together.' Yet this very combination forms the mainstay of many modern Western meals – steak and potatoes, hamburgers and chips, toast and eggs, spaghetti bolognese. The earliest recorded prohibition against this digestively noxious food combination appears in the Old Testament, when Jehovah instructs Moses to teach his people to eat their meat and bread at separate meals: 'At evening ye shall eat flesh, and in the morning ye shall be filled with bread.' In other words, bread and other starchy carbohydrates should be eaten for breakfast, without any meat, and meat should only be eaten for dinner in the evening, without bread. This advice accords exactly with the first law of trophology.

Simply by following this single cardinal rule, a primary source of acid indigestion and toxic putrefaction in the stomach and bowels is eliminated from the diet. Whenever meat, eggs or cheese are eaten together with bread, rice or other starch, the starch starts to digest in the mouth with secretions of the alkaline enzyme ptyalin, and this alkaline-forming digestive process continues when the starch reaches the stomach, blocking digestion of the protein by pepsin and hydrochloric acid, the other acid-forming enzymes required to digest animal proteins. Consequently, the alkaline requirements of starch digestion conflict in the stomach with the acid requirements of protein digestion, resulting in the digestion of neither and the fermentation and putrefaction of both. This in turn produces more toxins and acid wastes that further inhibit digestion and allow bacteria to gobble up all the available nutrients in the food and dump their own acid wastes into your digestive tract.

The second basic rule regarding consumption of animal proteins is: 'Don't combine two different kinds of animal protein at the same meal', such as meat and milk, eggs and cheese. This, too, is mentioned in the Bible and became known as the 'second Mosaic law' of diet, whereby Moses forbade his people to consume meat and milk together. This is sage advice in food combining, and has a sound scientific basis, since the strongest gastric enzyme activity on meat occurs during the first hour of digestion, whereas milk is digested mostly during the last hour, and eggs somewhere in between. Consequently, if two different types of animal protein are eaten together at the same meal, neither can be properly digested, and both putrefy instead. While it's fine to combine two types of meat, such as beef and chicken, or lamb and fish, tuna and prawns, no meat should be eaten together with milk, cheese or eggs.

Starchy carbohydrates
Starch is the carbohydrate culprit that causes acid indigestion, and since most carbohydrates eaten today are highly refined, their starch content is unnaturally elevated. Whole grains, which contain far less starch gram for gram than refined varieties, are easier to digest and combine much better with other foods, but anything that consists mainly of refined starch, such as white bread and pastries or white rice and noodles, should be eaten separately from all concentrated animal proteins such as meat, eggs and cheese.

Most people today eat starchy carbohydrates for breakfast, in the form of toast, porridge or cereal. Wholegrain versions of these foods are by far the better choice: they contain less starch, supply more vital nutrients than refined varieties and cause less severe acid-forming reactions when improperly combined with other foods. One of the worst breakfast combinations is packaged dry cereal made from factory processed grains, heavily sprinkled with refined white sugar and soaked in pasteurized cow's milk. Children suffer most from the ravages of this indigestible food combination, and it's a major factor in the obesity, constipation, skin problems and low resistance to disease which plague many of them today.

Since proper digestion of starch must begin in the mouth with thorough ensalivation by the ptyalin enzyme, it's important to chew all carbohydrate foods very well before swallowing, and not to drink any liquids with them. Any beverage taken together with starch dilutes the salivary secretions of ptyalin, preventing proper pre-digestion of starch in the mouth and resulting in fermentation in the stomach.

Fat

Fats such as butter and oil may be combined with most carbohydrates and all vegetables, but they should not be combined with concentrated animal proteins such as meat and eggs. Fat impairs the digestion of meat in the stomach by inhibiting the required gastric secretions. Consequently, for two to three hours after ingesting significant amounts of fat, levels of pepsin and hydrochloric acid in the stomach are sharply reduced, resulting in the putrefaction of any meat or eggs eaten along with the fat. You should therefore eat fats and proteins separately, or combine only very small amounts of one with normal portions of the other, and avoid eating 'marbled' meats such as bacon and fatty steaks.

Sugar

Refined white sugar is the single most acid-forming food substance in modern diets, and its presence in the stomach interferes with the proper digestion of almost all other foods. When sugary desserts or soft drinks are consumed at the same meal with meat, for example, the sugar blocks secretion of the gastric juices required to digest meat, resulting in putrefaction, fermentation and extreme acidity. When eaten with starchy carbohydrates, sugar shuts off salivary secretion of ptyalin in the mouth, and the starch lands in the stomach without the essential enzyme required to pre-digest it, resulting in fermentation and the production of acid wastes. To a lesser degree, sugar also causes fermentation and 'acid indigestion' when eaten with fruit and vegetables. Therefore, the best policy towards foods and beverages that contain a lot of refined sugar is not to combine them with proteins, starchy carbohydrates or any other category of food at the same meal. If you wish occasionally to indulge your 'sweet tooth' by eating ice cream, cakes, biscuits and other sweet confections made with refined sugar, it's best to eat them alone, preferably with some hot tea, and to flush the stomach with a glass or two of alkaline water an hour or two later.

Fruit

Fresh fruit is such a 'ripe' food that it requires virtually no digestion in the stomach. Instead, it moves quickly into the duodenum, where it dissolves and releases its nutrients for rapid assimilation. However, if its swift passage through the stomach is blocked by the presence of any other food, fruit gets delayed in the stomach, and its rich stores of natural sugars are immediately raided by the ever-present bacteria in the stomach. This causes everything in the stomach to quickly ferment, producing acids, generating gas and disrupting the entire digestive process. Melons and citrus fruits ferment even faster than other fruits and cause even worse gastric distress when combined with other foods, including other types of fruit, and should therefore not be eaten together with anything else.

If eaten in sufficient quantity and variety, fresh fruit can provide all the essential nutrients required for life, including amino acids, which are the basic building blocks of protein, as well as vitamins, minerals and active enzymes. Besides nourishing the body, fresh fruit also alkalizes the digestive tract, cleans the bloodstream and detoxifies the tissues. To obtain these benefits, however, fruit must be eaten by itself, not combined with other types of food, and while most fruits may be freely combined with each other, melons and citrus fruits should always be eaten by themselves, in strict accordance with the 'golden rule' of trophology: 'Eat it alone or leave it alone!'

Vegetables

Vegetables are the great common denominator in most equations of food combining. They combine very well with all proteins, including meat and eggs, as well as with starchy carbohydrates such as noodles, bread and rice, and also with fats. Vegetables assist digestion and assimilation of other foods by supplying essential minerals and enzymes that facilitate digestive functions. They also assist elimination by providing fibrous bulk to propel digestive wastes through the bowels, and most of them have strong alkaline-forming properties as well. Vegetables may therefore be eaten in unlimited quantities to complement meals based on either proteins or carbohydrates. The only food they don't combine well with is fruit.

When raw vegetables are eaten whole, as in salads, they can take a long time to digest and release their nutrients, owing to their high cellulose content. However, when extracted as pure juices, with the cellulose pulp removed, their nutritional value and alkalizing benefits increase significantly and are delivered more swiftly. The best way to eat fresh vegetables whole is to cook them very briefly by steaming, stir-frying or poaching, which softens the cellulose content sufficiently to allow easy digestion without destroying their nutritional value through prolonged exposure to heat.

Shortlist of alkaline- and acid-forming foods

In order to assist readers in learning how to compose harmoniously balanced meals based on the alkaline- and acid-forming properties of various foods, the chart below divides a wide

selection of common food items into alkaline and acid categories, and lists them in order of their relative strength. The
number next to each item indicates the *degree* of its alkaline-
or acid-forming effects, compared with the base number 1 for
the *least* alkalizing or acidifying item on the list. For example,
tofu is the least alkaline-forming food in the alkaline category
and therefore has a rating of 1. Strawberries, with a rating of
56, are 56 times more alkalizing than tofu, and ginger is 211
times stronger. Similarly, oysters are 80 times more acid-
forming than asparagus, but only slightly more acidifying than
salmon. This chart is based on information from Herman
Aihara's excellent booklet, *Acid and Alkaline*.

Acid-forming foods		*Alkaline-forming foods*	
rice bran	852	wakame seaweed	2608
bonita flakes	371	kombu seaweed	400
dried squid	296	ginger	211
dried fish	240	kidney beans	188
egg yolk	192	shitake mushrooms	175
oatmeal	178	spinach	156
brown rice	155	soya beans	102
tuna	153	bananas	88
octopus	128	chestnuts	83
chicken	104	adzuki beans	73
pearl barley	99	carrots	64
oysters	80	mushrooms	64
salmon	79	strawberries	56
buckwheat	77	potatoes	54
scallops	66	cabbage	49
pork	62	radishes	46
peanuts	54	squash	44
beef	50	sweet potatoes	43
cheese	43	turnips	42
abalone	36	orange juice	36

Acid-forming foods		Alkaline-forming foods	
whole barley	35	apples	34
prawns	32	egg white	32
peas	25	pears	26
beer	11	grape juice	23
bread	6	cucumbers	22
butter	4	watermelon	21
asparagus	1	aubergine	19
		coffee	19
		onions	17
		tea	16
		runner beans	11
		tofu	1

Live food for living people

It stands to reason that if 'dead food' hastens death, that 'live food' does the opposite and prolongs life. The rational choice for the retox diet is therefore to eat only live foods. The best definition of 'live food' was formulated back in the pre-junk food America of the 1930s by Dr E. V. McCullum, the pioneering nutritional scientist at Johns Hopkins University. His advice was this: 'Eat nothing unless it will spoil or rot, but eat it before it does!' That eliminates all processed and packaged foods produced with chemical preservatives, artificial flavours, synthetic dyes and other unnatural additives, as well as any food that has been highly refined, irradiated or genetically modified. Such food products are designed with only one purpose in mind: to extend the shelf life of the product. They do nothing to extend the life of the consumer.

One way to exclude dead food from your diet is to eat 40–50 per cent of your daily fare in the form of raw or very lightly cooked foods. Raw and rare cooked foods are only edible when fresh and complete with the essential elements of life, and this

natural freshness and vitality cannot be duplicated with the artificial flavours, chemical preservatives and other additives used
to produce processed foods. Live raw foods help clear the stagnation and eliminate the toxic debris produced in the digestive
tract by dead processed foods by supplying the active enzymes
and vital trace elements required to digest this inert toxic sludge,
and by providing fresh fibre bulk to dredge these wastes quickly
through the bowels and out of the body.

Another way to ensure there is life in the food you eat – as
well as in your own body – is to strictly eliminate all items from
your diet which contain chemical preservatives, dyes, flavouring
agents such as MSG, and any other non-nutritional additives.
Thousands of toxic chemicals, including some that are known
carcinogens, are commonly used to manufacture junk food, fast
food and other so-called convenience food. All of these synthetic
additives are extremely acid-forming and leave toxic residues
lodged in the tissues that are very difficult to excrete. This applies
equally to fresh produce grown with pesticides, herbicides and
chemical fertilizers, all of which contribute heavily to acidosis
and toxaemia. Although organically produced foods are more
expensive and difficult to find than factory farmed food, it's well
worth the extra cost and effort to eat only live natural foods that
are rich in nutrition and devoid of poisons. If the price of organic
foods is a bit 'rich' for your budget, the solution is to buy them
anyway, but to buy less. Eating just a small serving of organically grown, nutritionally complete food does more to nourish
the body and prolong life than eating a whole bushel of
processed factory food.

Last, but not least deadly, on the list of dead foods which
should be banished from your diet are the 'impostors': artificial
food substitutes that pose prettily on the supermarket shelves,
brightly packaged and labelled in order to catch your eye,
pretending to be healthy alternatives to real foods. Among the
worst offenders here are margarine, non-dairy creamer and all

other fake foods made from hydrogenated vegetable oils, as well as all synthetic sugar substitutes such as saccharin and aspartame. Not only are these fake foods dead, they were never alive to begin with, so they contain nothing whatsoever that supports life, and all of them wreak havoc with human metabolism. These phoney fat and sugar substitutes are all extremely acid-forming, extremely toxic to the tissues and, if consumed to excess, can also becomed very carcinogenic.

The CRON diet: calorie restriction/optimum nutrition

The CRON diet, which stands for calorie restriction/optimum nutrition, was developed as a means of extending the lifespan of any species by Dr Roy Walford, Biosphere veteran and author of *Beyond the 120 Year Diet*. Based on extensive long-term studies that Dr Walford conducted with rats, dogs and other mammal species, the CRON diet is designed to take advantage of the scientifically proven correlation between low calorie/high nutrient diets and longevity. The basic rationale for this direct link between the CRON diet and long lifespan is simple: maximum nutrition with minimum calories means maximum metabolic energy with minimum toxic waste. It also means that the body requires less energy to digest food and eliminate wastes, allowing more energy to be reserved for sustaining internal cleansing and immune functions. By reducing internal acidity and tissue toxicity to minimal levels while supplying optimum nutrition, the CRON diet counteracts the conditions which give rise to disease and degeneration, and provides the proper balance of essential elements and energy needed to support health and prolong life.

Traditional Chinese physicians have known about the life-prolonging benefits of calorie restriction for thousands of years, and their dietary prescription for health and longevity is succinctly summarized in the ancient dietary axiom to eat only *chi-ba fen bao*, or '70–80 per cent full'. Traditional Chinese cuisine was exquisitely well balanced to provide optimum nutrition, so the only dietary factor that required attention in Chinese food was quantity. The 'Chinese rule' to eat only until you're 70–80 per cent full is still a convenient measure for determining how much to eat at any meal, and knowing when to stop.

Another effective way to reduce the quantity of food eaten while also increasing its nutritional value is to chew, chew, chew your food until it's well enough masticated to dissolve in the mouth before swallowing. This is particularly helpful when eating carbohydrates, which require pre-digestion in the mouth in order to properly digest in the stomach. Chewing food well helps prevent the acid-forming reactions of putrefaction and fermentation in the stomach, increases assimilation of nutrients and reduces the transit time of digestive wastes through the bowels.

It's important to remember, however, that in order to effectively extend the human lifespan, both aspects of the CRON diet must be equally implemented – not just 'calorie restriction' but also 'optimum nutrition'. Following a low-calorie fad diet consisting mainly of denatured 'convenience' foods and eating them in indigestible combinations provides the body nothing but 'empty calories', and has the opposite effect by ruining health and shortening life. In the following pages, we'll take a brief look at several major categories of food commonly consumed in modern diets, and establish a few rational guidelines for determining which foods to include and which to eliminate when designing a new diet balanced for health and longevity.

Guide to eating mammals, birds and fish

In prehistoric times, when the human species still depended on meat to survive, people got their meat not at the supermarket but by killing mammals, birds and fish in the wilderness and eating them raw or slightly cooked the same day, fresh off the bone. Today, most humans still retain this primitive taste for the flesh of other species, even though meat products have become totally unnecessary and often very harmful factors in the human diet. Moreover, the meat that people get on their dinner plates today is a far cry from the fresh flesh of healthy wild animals which their ancestors ate.

The meat sold in markets today is loaded with powerful synthetic hormones and chemical steroids that are fed to livestock to stimulate rapid growth, increase weight and bring entire herds into heat simultaneously for breeding purposes. When humans eat this meat, the hormones are absorbed into their bodies and stimulate rapid growth in their tissues as well, and this has become a major contributing factor in the current widespread problem of obesity in the wealthy meat-eating countries of the West. These chemical growth stimulants and synthetic sex hormones also severely disrupt the delicate hormonal balances within the human body, especially in ovulating women and growing children. The extraordinarily high incidence of breast and cervical cancer, ovarian cysts and other reproductive disorders among women in the Western world is due in large part to the contamination of the human food chain with hormones and steroids fed to livestock in those countries.

Owing to the appalling conditions in which commercial livestock are raised, these animals must also be heavily dosed with antibiotics to keep them alive long enough to reach the slaughterhouse. Over 40 per cent of the antibiotics produced in the USA are fed directly to cattle, pigs, chickens and even to commercially farmed salmon and trout. Whoever who eats these products regularly receives a continuous infusion of powerful antiobiotic drugs that weakens their natural immune responses, kills all the friendly lactobacteria in the digestive tract and produces a state of chronic acidosis. In addition to all these toxic drugs and hormones, commercial livestock also assimilate all the poisonous pesticides, herbicides and chemical fertilizers used to grow the crops for their feed, and these toxins too pass into the body of the consumer. Anyone who wants to know more about the atrocious conditions livestock today suffer and how these hapless creatures are systematically drugged, poisoned and fed on dead, denatured food that often includes such delectables as sawdust, paper pulp and the processed cadavers of other animals that died of disease, should read John Robbins' latest book, *The Food Revolution*, and its prequel, *Diet for New America*. The conditions he describes prevail in the commercial meat industry throughout the world, not just in America, and anyone who still eats factory-farmed meat after reading either of these books has no one to blame but themselves for the consequences.

Even without all the toxic contamination in modern meat products, beef and pork have always been difficult for the human body to digest and process, and both are extremely acid-forming. The main problem is in the fat content: the type of fat in beef and pork fat inhibits gastric secretions in the stomach, clogs digestion and puts a huge strain on the liver, where all food fat must be processed. After conducting extensive studies in 16 countries, researchers in Canada established a close causal link between high consumption of pork products and cirrhosis of the liver, and in countries where pork is commonly consumed together with alcohol such as beer and wine, the incidence of cirrhosis soared to 1,000 times higher than average. Daily consumption of beef and pork can also establish the conditions that lead to the development of bowel cancer.

Other than wild game, which is almost impossible to get these days, the only red meat that is both beneficial to health and relatively safe to eat is lamb. Sheep generally graze in open pasture and get plenty of fresh air and natural sunlight, rather than being cooped up day and night in cages and pens and fed on dead industrial feed. It's still possible to buy lamb that has not been poisoned with drugs and steroids. Unlike the fat from cattle and pigs, lamb fat digests quite well in the human body, and it's a rich source of carnitine, an amino acid that transports fat into the cells for metabolism. Since the heart is the biggest burner of fat in the body, carnitine carries fat from the liver to fuel the heart, and this process, which can only be performed by carnitine, helps prevent cirrhosis and other liver damage caused by excess accumulation of fat in the liver. In the Himalayas, Middle East and Mediterranean regions, where lamb has always been the main meat food, arteriosclerosis, heart disease, bowel cancer and other ailments associated with high consumption of beef and pork are relatively rare.

When eating red meat, it's a good idea to cook it on the rare side, in order to preserve some of its enzymes to assist digestion and prevent damaging the proteins with excessive exposure to high heat. Using some strong mustard, horseradish or fresh ginger as a condiment for meat stimulates secretions of the gastric juices required to digest it.

As for poultry, the way chickens are produced for market today is even more of a horror story than pigs and cows. Up to 40,000 chickens are cooped up in steel cages in multi-storied 'poultry prisons', with two or three 'jail-birds' cramped into each cell, fed on dry pellets of noxious industrial feed laced with hormones and antibiotics. Anyone who wants to learn the whole ugly truth about this foul business is again referred to John Robbins' books.

Every year over 800 million chickens are killed in the UK for their meat. They are cooped up in steel cages in multi-storied 'poultry prisons' no bigger than an A4 sheet of paper. The chicks are selectively bred and pumped full of drugs to reach 'slaughter size' in just 41 days. Today's chickens are slaughtered when their eyes are still blue and they 'cheep' – in other words they are chicks in obese adult bodies. By the time they are killed, most of them are crippled as their legs cannot support their body weight. Could this possibly be a factor in the rampant obesity seen today among chicken-chomping children in America and other wealthy societies that adopt American fast-food diets? The average tissue mass of a typical chicken breast in America today is seven times greater than it was only 25 years ago. Again, one wonders what effects the hormones that produce these big-breasted chickens have on the breast tissues of women who eat those chickens.

Free-range chicken is certainly much safer to eat than 'jail-bird' chicken, but the term has become so abused by the commercial chicken industry that it's difficult to find a chicken these days that's been allowed to range freely in nature to forage for its own food. In many cases, the free range label only means that caged chickens are occasionally let out of their cells and allowed to 'range freely' around a fenced, concrete yard that's barren of vegetation, like convicts in a prison yard, then locked up again and fed the same denatured commercial feed that fully confined chickens eat. The only label designation that now assures you of getting a real chicken that's been naturally raised without drugs and other chemicals, is the term 'non-caged free-range chicken'. If you cannot find these genuine free rangers in your local markets, the only remaining options are to delete chicken from your diet, or else to raise them yourself.

If you wish to make flesh a regular part of your diet, the best choice is fresh seafood. Deep-water ocean fish such as tuna, swordfish and salmon are rich sources of essential fatty acids that cleanse the blood vessels of excess cholesterol and other fatty plaque deposits, dissolve clots and prevent sludging of red blood cells. These effects help prevent arteriosclerosis, heart attacks and strokes. Fresh seafood also supplies the essential minerals and trace elements from the sea that are required for balanced brain and nerve functions; that's why fish has long been known as 'brain food'. Frozen seafood is an equally good source of nutrition, as long as it's 'fresh frozen' soon after the catch and not processed in factories. Commercially farmed seafood, however, is not a good food choice. Like other commercial livestock, such as pigs and chickens, farmed fish are fed on industrially processed feed and heavily dosed with drugs and hormones, which pass into the body of the consumer when the fish is eaten. Similarly, unless you catch it yourself in a clean river or lake, freshwater fish is usually contaminated with the toxic pollutants that industry – particularly the commercial beef industry – dumps into public waterways.

Fat and oil

The first and foremost rule that governs healthy, rational choices in dietary fat and oil is this: strictly avoid *all* artificial substitutes for butter and cream, including margarine, shortening, non-dairy creamer and non-dairy whipped cream. All of these gummy, plasticine products are made with hydrogenated vegetable oils, which are forged at searing heats of over 225° C (500° F), then bubbled through with hydrogen and hardened with nickel. When natural fats are replaced in the diet with these artificially synthesized fats, the body incorporates them into the construction of new cells, which become defective and malfunction as a result. Since the cells of the brain and immune system require the most fat, these are the tissues which suffer the most damage from regular consumption of hydrogenated vegetable oil products. Here's how Dr Cass Igram, author of *Eat Right or Die Young*, describes the damage done to white blood cells and immune response when artificial fats made from hydrogenated oils are consumed:

> These cells incorporate the hydrogenated fats you eat into their membranes. When this happens, the white cells become sluggish in function, and their membranes actually become stiff. . . . This leaves the body wide

open to all sorts of derangements of the immune system. . . . In fact, one of the quickest ways to paralyze your immune system is to eat, on a daily basis, significant quantities of deep-fried foods, or fats such as margarine . . . [which] is associated with a greater incidence of a variety of cancers.

Real dairy butter, which is the *only* part of cow's milk that the human body can properly digest, is actually a rich source of metabolic energy, and if it comes from cows that are healthy and allowed to graze in green pastures, butter is an excellent dietary source of fat nutrition. *Ghee*, or clarified butter, is made by skimming off all the white protein particles from melted butter to produce a pure, clear 'butter oil'. This may be used for cooking at high heat without scorching the oil and producing free radicals. Fat rendered from beef (tallow) and pork (lard) should be eliminated entirely from the diet; both are highly acid-forming, extremely hard to digest and damaging to the liver.

The best overall choice in oil for cooking food, mixing dressings and other culinary purposes is high-grade olive oil. Olive oil can be used to cook food at high temperatures without producing an excess of free radicals, and it contains only the 'good fats', such as the mono-unsaturated variety. Other healthy choices in edible oils include sesame, sunflower, peanut (groundnut) and various other nut oils, preferably cold-pressed from organic sources. Many of the mass-produced, processed cooking oils found on supermarket shelves today, including corn, soya bean, rapeseed (canola), and the dubious blended vegetable oils, are not beneficial to human health, and some are downright hazardous, especially any that have been hydrogenated. To be sure, always read the label.

Dairy products

If health is the first priority when choosing foods for the human diet, then there are so many good reasons not to consume pasteurized cow's milk products from commercial dairies that it's difficult to understand why people who wish to stay healthy still do. Cow's milk contains 400 per cent more protein than human milk, including large amounts of cassein, a tough protein substance so strong and sticky that it's often used to make book binding glue and postal paste. Imagine what this stuff does to your bowels.

Pasteurization kills the active enzyme in milk that's required to digest it, and since most people don't produce this enzyme in their bodies, the milk stagnates in the stomach and the indigestible protein putrefies into a slimy sludge which oozes through the digestive tract and plasters gummy layers of mucus to the intestinal walls, forming a tough, rubbery lining that increasingly binds up the bowels. The reason that babies froth at the mouth and regurgitate foamy white phlegm after being fed pasteurized cow's milk is because their newly functioning stomachs, which are genetically designed to digest human milk, cannot digest the bovine cassein protein present in cow's milk.

Today, commercial dairy milk is rendered even more hazardous to human health by the high doses of synthetic hormones that are fed to dairy cows to make them produce more milk. Residues of these powerful hormones, which can force a cow's mammary glands to produce five to six times more milk than normal cows, enter the human system when this milk is consumed, and this can cause severe imbalances in the human endocrine system, especially in women and children. In recent years, family physicians throughout the USA have reported an alarming rise in premature puberty among girls as young as eight and nine, including full breast development, sexual fertility and pregnancy. Dairy hormones in the daily diet have become the major suspect in this abnormal development, and these hormones cause glandular deviations in adult women as well. In *Food and Healing*, nutritional therapist Annemarie Colbin writes, 'The consumption of dairy products, including milk, cheese, yoghurt and ice cream, appears to be strongly linked to various disorders of the female reproductive system, including ovarian tumours and cysts, vaginal discharges and infections.' In many cases, these problems quickly disappear after all dairy products are eliminated from the diet.

Women in the Western world are advised by their doctors to drink pasteurized cow's milk as a source of calcium to prevent osteoporosis, and yet the incidence of osteoporosis among dairy-consuming Western women continues to grow unabated. That's because the human body cannot assimilate the calcium in cow's milk; owing to its high phosphorus content, which blocks absorption of calcium in the bowels, cow's milk is definitely not a viable source of calcium for the human body. In fact, the acidity produced in the body by the putrefaction of milk products forces the body to leach calcium *out* of the body's own bones in order to restore alkaline balance in the bloodstream, and this only contributes further to osteoporosis. Doctors properly trained in basic nutritional science would never recommend cow's milk as a dietary source of calcium for human nutrition, especially when there are so many richer, more bio-available sources of dietary calcium than milk, none of which causes the digestive distress produced by processed dairy products and all of which deliver far more calcium. For example, while 100 g of cow's milk contains 118 mg of calcium, the same amount of almonds supplies 254 g, broccoli delivers 130 g, kale 187 g, sardines 400 g, kelp has a whopping 1,093 and 100 g of the humble sesame seed supplies a mega-dose of 1,160 mg of organic calcium to the body. So who needs cow's milk?

People who wish to include dairy items such as milk, cheese and yoghurt in their diets should choose products made from goat's milk, which has slightly alkalizing properties and contains the same basic proportions of protein, calcium, phosphorus and other nutrients as human milk. Since it contains very little fat, goat's milk is relatively easy to digest and is low in calories.

Grains

Most grains are warming, acid-forming yang foods and are best eaten with cooling, alkaline-forming vegetables to ensure digestive and metabolic balance. The only major food grain that's alkalizing is millet, which was the first grain to be cultivated as food in ancient China. Wheat, on the other hand, which has for centuries been the most popular grain food in the Western world, is one of the most highly acid-forming grains, and it can cause allergic reactions in people who consume it daily. Rye is a much better choice than wheat, especially for making bread, because it's less acid-forming, supplies more well balanced nutrition and rarely causes allergic reactions.

Grains are easier to digest and more nutritionally complete when consumed in whole form rather than refined. Whole grains are truly 'whole foods': they contain carbohydrates, proteins, fats, vitamins, minerals and fibre. Newcomers to the science of food combining often ask why a protein food such as meat and a carbohydrate food such as bread must be eaten separately in order to avoid indigestion and acidosis, whereas foods that contain both protein and carbohydrate, such as whole grains, may be eaten without causing trouble in the stomach. Dr Herbert Shelton, author of the booklet *Food Combining Made Easy*, answers this question as follows:

> There is a great difference between the digestion of a *food*, however complex its composition, and the digestion of a *mixture of different foods*. To a single article of food that is a starch-protein combination [e.g. whole

grains], the body can easily adjust its juices, both as to strength and timing, to the digestive requirements of the food. But when two foods are eaten with different, even opposite, digestive needs [e.g. meat and bread], this precise adjustment of juices to requirements becomes impossible.

When boiling grains in whole form as a staple food for meals, they should first be washed well, drained, then soaked in pure water for 2–3 hours, or overnight, before cooking. Alternatively, you may first toast the grains until golden brown in an oven or a dry pan over a medium-hot flame, prior to boiling. This toasting process, known as dextrinization, converts much of the starch content into simple sugars, making the cooked grain easier to digest and less acid-forming in the stomach. The chart below gives the cooking times, proportions of dry grain to water, and cooked yield for boiling brown rice, wild rice, buckwheat and bulgur:

Grain	Cooking time	Amount dry	Water	Cooked yield
brown rice	35–40 min.	1 cup	2 cups	2 ½ cups
wild rice	60 min.	1 cup	4 cups	3 ½ cups
buckwheat	20 min.	1 cup	5 cups	3 cups
bulgur	15 min.	1 cup	2 cups	2 ½ cups

The other way to prepare whole grains as food is to grind them into flour and bake bread. Bread is one of the most ancient and widely consumed foods in the Western world, but today virtually all of it is made with baker's yeast, which ruins much of the bread's nutritional value and causes allergic reactions in people who are sensitive to yeast. The problem with yeast as a leavening agent for bread is that it renders the calcium and magnesium in the flour insoluble and therefore unavailable to the body. Calcium and magnesium are the two most important

macro-minerals required for human health, and they play especially important roles in detox and alkaline balance. Whole grains
are one of the best dietary sources of these essential nutrients.
Even when high quality organically grown grains are used to
make bread, if the dough is leavened with yeast, it robs the body
of an important source of dietary calcium and magnesium, and
makes bread more acid-forming in the digestive tract.

The solution here is to 'go back to the basics' and eat only
wholegrain breads that are prepared with natural sourdough
leavening. Sourdough produces precisely the right balance of
pH and other vital factors that allow calcium, magnesium and
other minerals in wholegrain flours to become soluble during
digestion, which makes them easy to assimilate into the bloodstream. When Celtic sea salt is used in making sourdough bread,
it further increases the bread's bio-available magnesium content
and improves the fermentation of the dough, making the bread
even more digestible. Using sourdough cultures to ferment flour
for bread, pancakes and other leavened grain products is similar
to using lactobacteria to ferment milk and make yoghurt: the
bacteria pre-digests the protein and starch in the flour, rendering
it far easier to digest in the stomach.

Whenever eating grains, don't forget to chew well before
swallowing. This saturates the starch with ptyalin enzyme from
the salivary glands in the mouth, without which it cannot be
properly digested in the stomach. When grain foods are wolfed
down without sufficient mastication in the mouth, they ferment
rather than digest in the stomach, producing acid indigestion
and gas.

Fermented foods

Fermentation has been used as a way to prepare food for at least
as long as fire has, and fermented foods play an important role
in healthy human diets. Fermentation by 'friendly' bacteria

breaks down complex carbohydrates and proteins in food, pre-digesting them so that they are easier to digest and assimilate. Fermentation also increases the vitamin content in food, especially B vitamins, and provides abundant supplies of bio-active enzymes that assist digestion and help regulate pH balance in the digestive tract. The bacteria cultures used in fermented foods support the colonies of 'friendly' flora in the lower bowels, which facilitates regular bowel movements.

In Western diets, yoghurt and sauerkraut are good examples of fermented foods that provide both nutritional and digestive benefits. Traditional Asian cuisines feature a wide range of tasty, nourishing foods made by fermentation. Koreans eat a fiery fermented side dish called *kimchee*, made with cabbage, carrot, garlic and chilli at almost every meal. Thai dishes are liberally laced with a pungent fermented fish sauce called *namphla*, and Chinese cooks use lots of fermented soy sauce, chilli pastes, and beancurd products, and prepare a variety of fermented vegetable side dishes known as *pao-tsai*. Indonesians eat a delicious, nutrient-rich ferment of soya beans called *tempeh*, and Japanese cuisine features richly fermented *miso* paste for soups and sauces, fermented fish and vegetable side dishes, and the remarkably nutritious, strongly flavoured ferment of whole soya beans called *naddo*, which is one of the few non-animal dietary sources of vitamin B_{12}. All of these traditional Asian ferments of beans and vegetables are easier to digest and richer in nutritional value than commercial yoghurt made from pasteurized cow's milk, and are therefore the best choices in fermented foods.

'Sugar blues'

Sugar Blues is the title of a book by William Duffy, in which he states, 'The difference between sugar addiction and narcotic addiction is largely one of degree.' The average daily consumption per person of refined white sugar in America has reached an astounding 53 teaspoons, which amounts to about 225 g (8 oz) of sugar per person per day. This certainly qualifies as 'substance abuse', and such a high rate of sugar consumption definitely becomes addictive, causing symptoms similar to drug addiction.

Whenever such massive quantities of industrially refined sugar enter the body, the immune system treats it as a toxic substance, which it certainly is at those dosages, and this triggers a continuous auto-immune response that throws the whole system off balance. One of those emergency responses is the constant secretion of insulin from the pancreas, which is needed to break down the massive overdose of sugar in the bloodstream. Over time, this causes the pancreas to swell up from overstimulation, and finally to collapse from depletion, at which point diabetes develops. Meanwhile, the excess insulin activity in the bloodstream suppresses release of growth hormone in the pituitary gland, which weakens immune response and lowers resistance.

Refined sugar is one of the primary causes of obesity and arteriosclerosis in the Western world. When sugar is consumed to excess, the liver converts most of it into tryglycerides and stores it as fat, transforming the rest of it into the 'bad' cholesterol that gets deposited as a sticky sludge in the walls of the arteries. Sugar is also a primary cause of osteoporosis and tooth decay because the extreme acidosis it produces forces the body to re-alkalize itself by leaching calcium from bones and teeth.

That's not all. Excessive consumption of refined white sugar has extremely deleterious effects on human behaviour as well, particularly in children. The hyperactivity, learning disabilities and other behavioural disorders experienced by so many children today is largely due to excessive intake of sugar. Studies conducted by Dr C. Keith Connors at the Children's Hospital in Washington DC have established what he calls a 'deadly link' between excessive daily consumption of sugar – especially when combined with starch – and the development of hypertension, violent behaviour and learning impediments in children. In 1991, in order to reduce the exposure of children to this health hazard, Singapore banned the sale of all sugary, carbonated soft-drinks at schools and youth centres, setting off howls of protest from peddlers of the most popular and profitable brands of these addictive drinks. By contrast, many public schools in America sign exclusive contracts with the major producers of these acidifying, enervating, habit-forming drinks, in exchange for a cut of the profits, allowing children to freely nurse their sugar habits throughout the day from vending machines. Trial studies have shown that chronic violence among inmates in prisons drops dramatically when all foods made with refined sugar are withdrawn, and there's no reason to think that the same would not hold true for chronic violence in schools.

Artificial sweeteners such as saccharin and aspartame are every bit as bad for health as refined white sugar and should be just as strictly avoided, particularly in light of evidence linking these synthetic sweeteners with a wide range of disorders, including cancer. The best alternatives to refined white sugar are whole natural sweeteners such as unrefined raw cane sugar, honey and maple syrup. The latter is an especially good choice because it's a complete wholefood in itself, brimming with essential vitamins, minerals, trace elements and other nutritional factors drawn from deep within the earth by maple trees.

For weight-watchers and diabetics, nature provides the perfect herbal sweetener in the form of a plant called stevia. Stevia is extracted from the leaves of a shrub native to South America, and gram-for-gram it's 100 times sweeter than sugar. A serving the size of a match-head suffices to sweeten any hot or cold beverage, and it may also be used for sweetening porridge and for other culinary purposes. It also tastes good. Not only is stevia harmless to diabetics, it actually helps them by improving the efficiency of insulin activity in the bloodstream. Stevia is by far the most rational and healthy alternative to sugar for people who have a 'sweet tooth' but don't want to gain weight from all the extra calories in sugar, or who worry about developing diabetes from an excess consumption of refined white sugar. It's not expensive and, while not widely available in the UK, can be obtained from mail-order suppliers.

'The salt of life'

Like so many other fundamental foods, salt has been denatured by modern food processing methods and stripped of its most essential nutrients. The salt sold in supermarkets today for culinary and table use is over 99 per cent sodium chloride and, like refined white sugar, it's this industrially processed salt that's harmful to human health, not natural whole salt.

The most important element missing from refined salt is magnesium, a deficiency of which contributes to heart disease, nervous system disorders and immune deficiency. Clinical studies in Canada and the United States showed a dramatic decline in the mortality rate among heart-attack patients who were given intravenous injections of magnesium. In a 1997 study, UK researchers assessed the effects of a 24-hour infusion of magnesium in patients with unstable angina. Thirty-one received magnesium and 31 a placebo. After treatment, there were fewer ischaemia (inadequate supply of blood) episodes in the magnesium group and the duration of ischaemia in the placebo group was longer. Magnesium is also an essential supporting factor in phagocytosis, an important immune response whereby white blood cells destroy infectious bacteria and scavenge other pathogens in the body. Perhaps most important of all, magnesium regulates the balance of acid and alkaline elements in the cellular fluids, thereby keeping the biochemistry of the entire body properly balanced by automatically adjusting cellular pH levels. Dr Jacques de Langre, author of *Sea Salt's Hidden Powers*, cites magnesium as the single most vital element required to maintain proper pH balance in the body:

> The human organism functions at its peak only when the balance between acid and alkaline is maintained. All substances that nourish the body are either acid or alkaline. Magnesium possesses the remarkable ability to maintain the acid/alkaline balance within the organism.

The best source of magnesium and other essential minerals and trace elements is whole Celtic sea salt, as discussed in previous chapters. Celtic sea salt is only 87 per cent sodium chloride, plus it contains the full spectrum of 81 other macro-and micro-minerals from the sea, all in precisely the proportions required by the human body. Those who wish to increase their intake of magnesium in order to correct blood acidosis and alkalize the cellular fluids may use the fluid bittern of Celtic sea salt, or the liquid blend of magnesium chloride and Celtic sea salt, mentioned in Chapter 2 on page 50.

Super supplements

Debate continues to rage regarding the efficacy of vitamins and other concentrated nutritional supplements and, like most health issues, both sides have their valid points. For one thing, there's a big difference between the benefits of synthetically manufactured supplements and those extracted from natural sources without the use of heat or industrial solvents. The efficacy of any supplement also depends to a great extent on other supporting factors, such as diet, consistent dosage, use of medical and recreational drugs, exercise and overall lifestyle. One thing can be said for certain: even the very best supplements cannot compensate for the ill effects of poor diet, malnutrition, excessive smoking and drinking, frequent use of pharmaceutical drugs and a high-stress lifestyle. Unless you're willing to systematically adjust all the basic factors of life, there's no point going to the expense and trouble of using costly supplements.

The supplements recommended below are all derived from natural sources, and each provides specific forms of protection against various factors which contribute to acidosis and toxaemia. While some of these supplements also have excellent nutritional benefits, the primary reason for their inclusion here is their facilitating role in daily detox functions: all of them have potent alkalizing, detoxifying and digestive properties which assist in the elimination of toxins and acid wastes from the tissues and continuously purify the bloodstream, thereby helping to keep the whole system properly balanced.

Antioxidants

Antioxidants scavenge and neutralize free radicals, which are highly reactive molecular fragments produced internally by natural metabolic processes as well as by pollutants assimilated from external sources, such as contaminants in food, water and air. Free radicals are the 'cellular terrorists' of the body, roaming randomly through the tissues, blasting holes in cell walls, damaging DNA codes, disrupting vital functions and laying waste to the internal terrain of the body. Antioxidants are the special 'commandos' introduced into the body with food, water and air to hunt down free radicals and terminate their destructive activity. With the steep rise in free radical activity today caused by toxic contamination within the body, antioxidants have become one of our strongest allies in the ongoing war against the 'cellular terrorism' of free radicals.

Certain nutrients, such as vitamins C, E and betacarotene, and the minerals zinc and selenium, play key roles in the body's antioxidant defences. Vitamin E breaks the self-generating chain-reactions whereby free radicals operate, and boosts the body's overall immunity and resistance. Vitamin E also helps protect the tissues against damage from toxic chemicals, such as mercury, lead, benzene and other poisons, and has an inhibiting effect against the development of cancer and heart disease. Vitamin C effectively scavenges a wide range of free radicals and works within the cells as well to protect DNA from free radical damage. It also provides specific protection against cardiovascular disease and enhances overall immune response. Betacarotene is the strongest antioxidant for scavenging an extremely reactive type of free radical known as singlet oxygen, and it also inhibits formation of cancerous tumours.

Selenium is a trace element that has been almost totally leached out of the food chain by modern farming and food processing methods. Selenium is essential for the synthesis of peroxidase, one of the body's most important antioxidant enzymes, which neutralizes hydrogen peroxide and other peroxide radicals produced in the body by fats. Selenium itself bonds with mercury, lead, cadmium and arsenic, neutralizing these heavy toxins and carrying them away for excretion. Selenium has become so scarce in food that supplementary supplies are the only viable source for most people today. Zinc is the key element in the body's other major antioxidant enzyme, superoxide dismutase (SOD), which scavenges free radicals in all of the body's tissues and vital fluids.

Whatever other vitamin and mineral supplements you may wish to take as part of your daily diet, it's definitely a good idea to include therapeutic doses of vitamins E, C and betacarotene, plus the minerals selenium and zinc, in order to ensure sufficient antioxidant activity, especially if you live in a polluted urban environment.

Recent studies in Japan, China and America have shown that unfermented green tea from Japan and semi-fermented High Mountain Oolung Tea from Taiwan have very potent anti-oxidant properties and provide significant protection against cancer. While both green tea and High Mountain Oolung have strong anti-oxidant activity, the amount of green tea needed to be drunk in order to have a therapeutic effect can irritate the stomach, and it's not nearly as fragrant and flavoursome as the top grades of High Mountain Oolung Tea from Taiwan, which may be consumed freely throughout the day without upsetting the stomach.

The anti-cancer effect of green and High Mountain Oolung tea is produced by compounds known as polyphenols, and research in Japan has demonstrated that High Mountain Oolung provides particularly strong protection against toxic damage and cancer formation in the lungs. In East Asia, where people smoke heavily, High Mountain Oolung has long been the tea of choice among smokers, and those who drink it daily have a consistently lower incidence of lung cancer than smokers who don't. One of the ways in which this tea suppresses growth of cancerous tumours is by inhibiting angiogenesis, a process whereby tumours generate growth of their own blood vessels to allow them to expand and multiply. Green and High Mountain Oolung teas also contain half a dozen types of catechins, which are potent phytochemicals that strengthen antioxidant defences by stimulating production of peroxidase, SOD and other important antioxidant enzymes in the body. On top of all that, these teas aid digestion, alkalize bodily fluids, purify the bloodstream and gently stimulate the nervous system without racing the heart, as coffee does.

Another primary source of antioxidant defence in the body is negative ions derived from ionized air and water, and the best way to enlist this ally into your army of antioxidants is to drink ionized water and breathe ionized air, as discussed in previous chapters.

Green food
Green food has already been mentioned in Chapter 5 as a potent cleansing supplement for detox diets, but it's also very useful as

a source of essential nutrients and blood purifiers. Green food's strong alkalizing and internal cleansing properties make it an excellent supplement for counteracting the internal pollution and acidity produced in the body by modern diets and eating habits, and its full-spectrum profile of essential nutrients compensates for common nutritional deficiencies, ensuring the body a daily supply of all the vital elements it needs to function properly.

Enzymes

Enzymes are the 'spark plugs' of human metabolism, providing the ignition that catalyzes every metabolic reaction in the body. Over 5,000 different enzymes have so far been identified in the human body, and without them the whole system would grind to a halt. Here's how Dr Edward Howell, one of the world's foremost authorities on enzymes, describes their importance in his book *Enzyme Nutrition:*

> No mineral, vitamin or hormone can do any work without enzymes. Our bodies, all of our organs, tissues and cells, are run by metabolic enzymes. They are the manual workers that build our bodies from proteins, carbohydrates and fats.

Among the thousands of enzymes in the body, the three most important types for detox and cleansing purposes are antioxidant enzymes, such as peroxidase and SOD, digestive enzymes, such as those secreted by the pancreas to handle the advanced stages of digestion, and food enzymes, which are not produced in the body and can only be obtained from fresh raw foods. Food enzymes, which are destroyed by heat in cooking and by chemical additives in processed foods, are required for the first stages of digestion in the stomach and, if they are missing, complex foods such as proteins and carbohydrates cannot be completely digested. Unless your daily diet consists of at least 30–50 per cent fresh, enzyme-rich raw foods, you should take capsules of food enzymes with all meals that consist mainly of cooked foods. The four primary food enzymes required for digestion are as follows:

Protease This enzyme digests protein as well as pathogenic bacteria, damaged cells, the membranes around viruses, inflammatory fluids such as pus and phlegm, and any other harmful substance that contains protein.

Amylase Amylase digests carbohydrates in food and helps dissolve pus and phlegm in damaged tissues. Combined with lipase, amylase digests a wide range of viruses and helps eliminate impacted mucus from inflamed lungs and bronchial passages.

Lipase This is the enzyme responsible for digesting fats. It also dissolves the fatty part of the membrane that envelops many types of virus, and the fatty deposits in the arteries.

Cellulase Cellulase digests the cellulose content in food, so that it may pass easily through the digestive tract as fibrous bulk to assist the elimination of wastes.

Food enzymes have strong alkaline-forming properties, which help reduce acid-forming reactions throughout the digestive tract and prevent blood acidosis. Because they improve digestive efficiency, food enzymes also reduce production of toxic wastes in the digestive tract, thereby preventing the development of toxaemia. In addition to taking them for digestive purposes with cooked meals, food enzymes may also be taken on an empty stomach when ill, in which case they enter general circulation in the bloodstream, assisting other immune factors such as white blood cells on 'search and destroy' missions against pathogens and pollutants and breaking down mucus, phlegm and pus in ailing organs and damaged tissues.

Supplements containing both digestive enzymes and food enzymes are available in tablet or capsule form for convenient daily use.

'Alka-aid'

In case of sudden gastrointestinal distress caused by excess acidity from wrong food combinations, highly acid-forming food such as sugar and meat, excessive use of pharmaceutical or recreational drugs, or intake of poisonous substances, the following supplements may be taken for fast, effective alkalization in the stomach and digestive tract. All of them are natural products and perfectly safe to use, and you may take more than one at a time for even stronger alkalizing effects.

Fresh lemon juice Mix the juice of one large or two small fresh lemons (not limes) with 100 ml water, and take 1 teaspoon every 15–20 minutes until the acid crisis passes. This is a particularly effective therapy for kidney stones.

Apple cider vinegar A great stomach alkalizer and digestive aid, apple cider vinegar contains malic acid, not the acidifying acetic acid found in other vinegars. It increases the flow of gastric juices in the stomach and counteracts acidity throughout the digestive tract. As a digestive aid, take 2 tablespoons with 1 teaspoon of honey in warm water, 20–30 minutes before meals; or take it any time of day or night on an empty stomach for swift alkaline relief.

Cream of tartar A highly alkalizing source of natural potassium, ½ teaspoon of cream of tartar may be stirred into 50 ml or so of water and taken for immediate relief of acid-forming reactions in the body, including the acidity produced by stress and anxiety.

Charcoal powder Pure powdered charcoal in capsule or tablet form may be used in cases of extreme stomach acidity due to food poisoning, fermentation and putrefaction, or poor digestion. Take 4–5 capsules, or stir 1 teaspoon of the powder into a glass of water, for quick symptomatic relief of strong acid reactions in the stomach.

Bicarbonate of soda Sodium bicarbonate swiftly neutralizes almost any sort of excess acidity in the stomach, and it may be used as often as required for such relief. Take 1 level teaspoon stirred into a glass of water, and repeat again later if necessary.

Shortlist of suggestions for cultivating rational eating habits

Many people these days prefer having important new information on healthy lifestyle habits succinctly summarized in list format, so they can tack it to the kitchen cupboard or family bulletin board for quick and easy daily reference. The dozen dietary precepts listed below may serve this purpose:

1. Don't eat unless you're hungry, and when you do eat, follow the 'Chinese Rule' of eating only *chi-ba fen bao*, '70–80 per cent full'.
2. Whether cooking food at home or ordering it in a restaurant, keep your meals as simple as possible by not combining more than three or four different categories of food at the same meal, and by combining those properly in accordance with the laws of trophology.
3. Strictly avoid eating all products made with hydrogenated vegetable oils.
4. In addition to balancing your individual meals by the rules of food combining, balance your whole diet according to season and climate: in the heat of summer, eat more cooling fresh vegetables and fruit; in the cold of winter, eat more warming proteins and carbohydrates; and always try to eat food that's in season.
5. Try to eat at least 30–50 per cent of your daily diet in the form of fresh raw foods – more in summer, less in winter.
6. Strictly avoid consuming any form of artificial sweeteners, and strictly limit intake of refined white sugar. If you like sweet things and are worried about calories or diabetes, use natural stevia as your sweetener.

7. Try to chew your food 30–40 times before swallowing, especially when eating starchy carbohydrates. Brown rice, which is acid-forming, actually becomes alkaline-forming if chewed at least 100 times, due to abundant ensalivation with the alkaline enzyme ptyalin in the mouth. You may not wish to chew all bread, rice and noodles that many times, but at least be aware that the more you chew it, the further it moves towards the alkaline side of the scale, and the less acidity it produces in the stomach.

8. Don't drink juice or water together with your meals because it dilutes salivary and gastric secretions, which delays digestion and permits fermentation. A glass of beer or wine sipped slowly with meals is fine, because beer and wine are fermented beverages, which means they are 'pre-digested' and contain enzymes that assist digestion in the stomach; hence the old saying, 'Take a little wine for the stomach's sake'.

9. Do try to drink at least six glasses (1.5 litres) of pure, alkaline water every day, but drink it only between meals. A good regimen is to drink two glasses immediately upon arising in the morning; one glass late morning, before lunch; another two glasses in the afternoon between lunch and dinner; and one final glass between dinner and bedtime.

10. Eat the sort of food that fits your lifestyle and work habits. Unless you do hard manual labour every day, or engage in strenuous physical exercise, don't eat too much animal protein and fat, because most of it will rot in your bowels and poison your body with toxic by-products of putrefaction, rather than being used to build new muscle and connective tissue. If you do a lot of mental work, eat plenty of complex whole carbohydrates to provide sustained cerebral energy, but take it easy on refined sugar and starch. 'You are what you eat', and therefore you should eat to suit the way you are.

11. Eat your meals only when you can take the time to sit down, relax and eat properly; don't eat in a hurry or 'on the run'. The faster you eat food, the slower it digests.

12. Do not eat solid food when you're sick, especially when you have a fever or chills, or when you feel acute pain. And don't eat when you're feeling emotionally upset or mentally unbalanced, such as when you're angry, anxious, worried or confused; the digestive system shuts down under these conditions, so whatever enters the stomach just sits there and decays, forming acids and toxins, which only makes your condition worse. Fasting is the best cure for most ills.

Last but not least, always try to follow the 'golden mean' of moderation in food. An ancient Chinese adage states, 'Disease enters the body through the mouth', and this dietary wisdom is echoed in a similar Western maxim, 'We dig our graves with our teeth'.

Towards the end of the 19th century, a group of scientists spent the better part of a decade travelling through Europe, Scandanavia and the British Isles, searching out and investigating as many cases as they could find of individuals who had already lived past the age of 100 and were still alive. Altogether they located nearly 2,000 living centenarians, some of whom were already well past 150 and on their way to becoming bi-centenarians. After carefully questioning these venerable elders and their families regarding their personal lifestyles and daily eating habits, the common factor discovered in all cases was moderation in food. Here's an excerpt from their report, as quoted in Dr Theodore Baroody's book *Alkalize or Die*:

> On reviewing nearly 2,000 reported cases of persons who lived more than a century, we generally find some peculiarity of diet or habits to account for their alleged longevity; we find some were living amongst all the

luxuries . . . others in the most abject poverty . . . some drank large quantities of water, others little; some were total abstainers from alcoholic drinks, others drunkards; some smoked tobacco, others did not; some lived entirely on vegetables, others to a great extent on animal foods . . . some worked with their brains, others with their hands; some ate one meal a day, others four or five . . . in fact, we notice a great divergence both in habits and diet, but in those cases where we have been able to obtain a reliable account of the diet, we find **one great cause** which accounts for the majority of cases of longevity: **moderation in the quantity of food.**

Let's leave the final word on this topic to the ancient Greek philosopher Diogenes, who left us much sage advice regarding the foibles and follies of human behaviour: 'As houses well stored with provisions are likely to be full of mice, so the bodies of those who eat much are full of diseases.'

CHAPTER 12

Advice on Smoking and Drinking

Smoking and drinking are the most common and widespread forms of so-called 'recreational drug use' throughout the world today. If we're going to discuss these issues rationally within the context of human health and longevity, then we must be perfectly clear about two basic points. The first is the fact that tobacco and alcohol are potent, habit-forming drugs, and smoking and drinking are essentially methods of delivering these drugs into the human system. Most people who use tobacco and alcohol daily wince when reminded that these substances are 'drugs', and many of them deny it on the assumption that because tobacco and alcohol are legal and don't require a prescription, they are neither drugs nor dangerous. This is wishful thinking, and anyone who smokes or drinks on that basis tends not to exercise the caution and self-discipline that should govern the use of any potent drug.

The second point we must bear in mind here is this: the distinction people make between 'recreational' and 'therapeutic' use of drugs, including tobacco and alcohol, is tenuous at best, and the difference between the 'recreational' and 'therapeutic' effects of a particular drug is usually more a matter of semantics than substance. Pray tell: who's to say whether a woman sitting in a café and lighting up her third cigarette over the same cup of coffee is smoking 'like a chimney' because it's so much fun and tastes so good ('recreational'), or because it instantly relieves her tension, calms her nerves and helps her think more clearly ('therapeutic')? And who can tell whether a man drinking his third martini during 'happy hour' at his favourite bar after work is doing so as a friendly social gesture and an epicurean experience ('recreational'), or as a quick-fix remedy for stress, anxiety or depression ('therapeutic')?

From the viewpoint of health, it doesn't matter whether the reason people smoke or drink is recreational or therapeutic, because the basic effects they have on the body and mind are the same either way. Both tobacco and alcohol belong to a class of drugs known as intoxicants and, as the name clearly indicates, they are not only in*toxic*ating but also toxic. The reason that people take such drugs, despite the fact that they are toxic to the body, is because a side effect of these substances is to intoxicate the mind. All intoxicants have a strong natural affinity for brain and nerve tissues, and the 'high' (or 'low') which they produce in the mind is a direct result of their toxic effects on brain and nerve cells; that's why this psycho-active effect is known as in*toxic*ation. By altering the body's brain chemistry and interfering with nerve transmissions, intoxicants change the way the mind experiences the world through the body's physical senses, thereby producing an 'altered state of mind'. People who use intoxicants do so because the way they normally experience the world causes them to feel pain, anger, sadness, fear or anxiety, and they know that they can alter these unhappy feelings instantly with a quick nip of whatever 'turns them on'.

Among the many intoxicants found in nature, modern societies have chosen, for reasons that we shall not speculate upon here, to make tobacco and alcohol the primary and only legal forms of recreational drugs. The point remains, however, that like all toxic substances which have intoxicating side effects on the mind – including some of the most potent medicinal plants and minerals in traditional herbal medicine – tobacco and alcohol also have very specific physiological effects in the body, and these effects can be used beneficially as therapy for relieving the symptoms of various ailments and correcting internal imbalances, particularly in the nervous system. Therefore, like all toxic substances that have both therapeutic and recreational applications, tobacco and alcohol should always be used with caution and moderation to ensure that the user enjoys the benefits of the desired effects, regardless whether they are used mainly for 'recreational' or 'therapeutic' purposes, without causing serious toxic damage to the body.

'Smoke signals'

From the point of view of health, the best advice on smoking is this: Don't smoke!

While not every substance that's smoked is addictive, smoking itself is highly habit-forming, and while some smokes may be marginally more harmful than others, the real damage to health is caused by smoking itself, not by the particular substance smoked. Smoking involves the inhalation of highly toxic by-products of combustion, many of which are carcinogenic. 'Where there's smoke there's fire', and when fire burns dried plant material such as tobacco, not only does it produce searing hot smoke, it also produces extremely poisonous chemicals that damage the delicate lining of the bronchia and lungs, cause highly acid-forming reactions in the blood and leave harmful toxic residues in the tissues. So unless you have more than recreational reasons for smoking, it's simply not worth the risk.

Nevertheless, all kinds of people throughout the world choose to smoke and, like everything else in life, there are relatively good ways and bad ways to conduct a smoking habit, especially for those who smoke primarily as a means of balancing the nervous system and stimulating cerebral functions. During the

1950s, the renowned clairvoyant healer Edgar Cayce sometimes advised clients to smoke 3–8 cigarettes of tobacco per day to control the symptoms of nervous disorders and compensate for inherent imbalances in their neurochemistry. It didn't matter whether the client already smoked or not, but Cayce stipulated that in order to gain the desired therapeutic effects without harming health, it was essential not to exceed his recommended daily dosage of 3–8 cigarettes. Tobacco is a potent medicinal herb with strong natural affinity for brain and nerve tissues. Even in very moderate doses such as those recommended by Cayce, tobacco stimulates abundant secretions of a wide range of vital neurotransmitters that are essential for balanced brain functions. In Cayce's time, cigarettes were not yet contaminated with dioxin and the hundreds of other carcinogenic chemicals that are used to manufacture cigarettes today, so they were still a relatively safe product, especially when used according to Cayce's guidelines. For people who cannot think clearly or function properly in society due to nervous disorders caused by inherent or acquired imbalances in their neurochemistry, the moderate risks to health posed by smoking 3–8 cigarettes made with pure tobacco and rolled in chemical-free paper are certainly acceptable, if that's what it takes to control their symptoms. As long as smokers don't exceed such a moderate daily dosage, they can gain significant therapeutic benefits from smoking tobacco, at minimum cost to health, and the smoking habit can become more helpful than harmful.

Similarly, many people today suffering from the advanced stages of cancer and AIDS report that smoking a bit of cannabis hemp stimulates their appetites and restores their capacity to digest food and assimilate nutrition, while also relieving the intense physical pain caused by their conditions and allowing them to sleep soundly at night. Prior to its prohibition, opium was also smoked as much for its medicinal benefits as for pleasure. In fact, during the 18th and 19th centuries in China, traditional doctors often recommended that elderly people suffering from chronic pain and incurable degenerative conditions associated with ageing start smoking opium in moderate daily dosages in order to control their discomfort and permit them to continue enjoying life. While certainly addictive, opium is no more so than tobacco, and smoking opium is considerably less harmful to health than smoking either tobacco or hemp, as evidenced by the remarkable longevity of many old Chinese opium smokers who properly conducted their habits and never exceeded their daily measure.

Today, however, both opium and hemp are prohibited, and tobacco is the only neuro-active medicinal herb that may be smoked legally for recreational or therapeutic purposes. Smokers should be aware, however, that tobacco is at least as addictive as opium, and that it's an even more difficult addiction to break than opiates; smoking tobacco is also more hazardous to health than smoking either hemp or opium. Nevertheless, since tobacco remains the only legal and socially condoned form of smoking throughout most of the world today, we shall limit our discussion here to tobacco.

Cigarettes

If you smoke cigarettes, the best advice is not to exceed Edgar Cayce's recommended daily allowance of 3–8 cigarettes, and to strictly follow this cardinal rule: Roll your own, or leave them alone! Factory-made cigarettes today truly live up to their designation as 'coffin nails', but what causes lung cancer and eventually kills the smoker is not the tobacco – it's the carcinogenic chemicals added to the tobacco and the paper in the cigarette production process. Among the approximately 2,000 toxic chemicals commonly found in commercially produced cigarettes today, dioxin poses the greatest threat to human health. Dioxin is a proven carcinogen that not only causes cancer but also produces genetic mutations, reproductive defects and brain damage. According to the Environmental Protection Agency in America, 'dioxin is by far the most toxic chemical known to mankind', and a report issued by a group of distinguished German scientists in 1998 concludes that dioxin alone is responsible for at least 12 per cent of all human cancers in industrialized societies. A UK study published in 1998 made it clear that dioxin can cause breast cancer in rats. The researchers exposed pregnant rats to small amounts of dioxin on the 15th day of pregnancy; the female offspring of the dioxin-exposed rats were born normal, but by the time they were seven weeks old, their mammary glands had developed an unusually high number of 'terminal end buds' – the places in the breast where cancers develop. This is definitely not something you want to inhale from the burning tip of a cigarette – not unless you're trying to kill yourself.

Many popular brands of cigarette today also contain radioactive residues from the uranium dust which commercial growers add to the chemical fertilizers they use on their tobacco crops. Why on earth they add radioactive material to the soil in which tobacco is grown has not been explained, but traces of radioactive isotopes of uranium are present in their products as well as in the lungs of people who smoke them. No wonder the Marlboro Man succumbed to lung cancer at the height of his fame.

The paper used to manufacture ready-made cigarettes is even more contaminated with poisonous chemicals than the tobacco itself. Cigarette smokers who are still reluctant to take the time to roll their own cigarettes should try this experiment: cut open a typical popular brand of cigarette, remove the tobacco, flatten out the paper, and lay it in an ashtray; with the glowing tip of a lit cigarette, touch one corner of the paper and observe what happens. The edge of the paper ignites and the entire sheet gradually incinerates to ash, without bursting into flame, with the glowing edge fizzling and sparkling like the fuse of a firecracker as it eats its way through the paper until it's gone. The chemicals added to cigarette paper to produce this effect are similar to those used in making fuses for firecrackers and other explosives, and the reason they're added is to make sure that the cigarette continues burning even when the smoker isn't puffing on it, in order to increase consumption and sales of cigarettes. Smokers accustomed to the convenience of ready-made factory cigarettes may find rolling their own a chore at first, but it's not nearly as inconvenient as getting lung cancer. Here again, if health and longevity are important considerations, the 'cost/ benefit' ratio of smoking 'coffin nails' compared with that of rolling your own cigarettes clearly dictates that you roll your own.

Good quality, organically grown tobaccos that are free of chemical additives and radioactive residues are now available on the market, and while they may be somewhat more expensive than commercial factory brands, if you roll your own cigarettes and smoke moderately, your consumption will decline so much that it offsets the extra cost of buying pure tobacco. It's equally important to use pure cigarette papers that have not been chemically treated to make them burn faster, and these too are readily available in tobacco shops. One of the purest cigarette papers is Club brand, made by S. D. Modiano of Italy. These have no gum or glue and are thin as a butterfly's wing, yielding a minimum of toxic wastes when burned.

Cigars

'A woman is just a woman,' wrote Kipling, 'but a cigar is a smoke!' While this doesn't say much for Kipling's feelings towards women, it says a lot about the way dedicated cigar smokers feel about their preferred manner of smoking tobacco. Cigars rolled in natural whole tobacco leaves were the first form of smoking brought to England and Europe from the New World, and purists still feel that only a cigar is a real 'smoke'. Paper-rolled cigarettes were a later British and European development, which then replaced cigars as the world's most widespread form of tobacco smoking.

Assuming that they are made from pure tobacco uncontaminated by chemical additives and rolled in natural leaf, cigars are significantly less hazardous to human health than cigarettes. Former President Clinton's claim not to have inhaled marijuana may be fatuous, but he probably didn't inhale the smoke from his cigars. Cigars are designed to allow nicotine to be gradually absorbed through the mucous membranes in the mouth and nasal cavities, as smoke wafts continuously through the lips and nostrils, without inhaling it into the lungs. Since it takes much longer to smoke a cigar than a cigarette, by the time the smoker has finished the cigar, he (or she) will have slowly but surely assimilated enough nicotine into the bloodstream to suffice the body's requirements for quite some time. To obtain therapeutic dosages of nicotine from cigarettes, the smoke must be inhaled all the way through the bronchia and into the lungs, a much more invasive way of smoking that damages the delicate lining of these organs with heat and carcinogenic chemicals. While good cigars made by hand with pure tobacco, such as the better brands produced in Cuba, are far more expensive than commercially produced brands, the latter are every bit as hazardous to health as factory-made cigarettes owing to the toxic chemical additives and synthetic wrappers used to mass-produce them. The extra cost of a pure cigar may therefore be offset in exactly the same way as the extra cost of pure cigarette tobacco and pure food – consume less, and enjoy it more!

Pipes

The third way to smoke tobacco is to use a pipe. Here, too, only pure tobacco that's free of chemical additives and artificial flavourings agents, should be smoked in pipes. Owing to growing awareness among smokers regarding the deadly dangers of chemical contaminants in tobacco, many tobacco shops these days stock a variety of organically grown pipe tobaccos flavoured only with natural plant essences. Besides ordinary tobacco pipes, water pipes may also be used to provide an additional measure of protection against the harsh by-products of combustion by running the smoke through water first.

'Fire water'

'Fire water' is the term which native American tribes used to describe the rum and other liquors brought to North America by British and European colonists. Alcohol intoxication contributed heavily to the downfall of traditional tribal cultures in North America, just as it did in Australia when British settlers introduced 'devil rum' to the indigenous aboriginal tribes there. The blood, liver and brain chemistry of these genetic groups are unable to properly metabolize alcohol, resulting in devastating destructive effects on their bodies and minds whenever it is consumed. For this reason, alcohol still remains a 'forbidden fruit' in many traditional tribal cultures, as well as in most Islamic countries and many parts of India, where its consumption is strictly prohibited and severely punished.

In the Western world, however, from early Greek and Roman times to the present day, alcohol has always been the main intoxicant of choice, and liquor is consumed in more variety and volume than anywhere else on earth. When Westerners began to colonize parts of Asia during the 17th and 18th centuries, they brought their liquor and drinking habits with them, prompting native observers to remark, 'Liquor is to the white man as mother's milk is to babies'.

From the viewpoint of traditional Eastern medicine, 'fire water' is actually a very apt term for alcohol. When alcohol is metabolized, it produces a lot of heat in the body, and if consumed daily in large amounts, this constant metabolic 'fire' tends to 'burn out' the internal organs, particularly the liver and brain. Alcohol is also a potent solvent of organic matter, which means it can dissolve organic tissue such as brain and liver cells, and its metabolism in the body is extremely acid-forming. As previously noted, high acidity is also regarded as a condition of yang excess, so drinking 'fire water' produces extremely yang conditions of 'fire-energy excess' both as excess heat and excess acidity.

The first drink or two of any liquor has a swift stimulating effect on human metabolism, producing a fast flush of body heat and a big surge of extra physical and mental energy. However, if the drinker continues to drink, the excess acidity and toxic waste produced in the blood and tissues by the continuous metabolism of alcohol accumulate rapidly, overloading the system with toxic metabolites and rapidly depleting reserves of vital nutrients and energy. As the body struggles to process and excrete the toxins and quell the metabolic 'fire' more alcohol enters the bloodstream with each sip, adding more fuel to the fire and progressively weakening the body's vital functions. At the same time, the intoxication produced in the mind as a side effect of the toxic influence of alcohol on brain and nerve tissues continues to grow more intense with each drink, disorienting the drinker's mind and producing a drunken stupor that ends in loss of consciousness. The toxic metabolite of alcohol which causes the most damage to brain and nerve cells, and which destroys liver tissue, is acetaldehyde. This highly reactive, extremely toxic acid poisons the bloodstream and corrodes the cells and tissues. Crude cheap liquor, which produces far more of this toxic acid waste in the body than more refined forms of alcohol, is known among derelict drinkers as 'rot-gut' because of the highly corrosive effects of this compound on the internal organs.

Contrary to popular notions, the forms of alcohol that are most hazardous to human health are not 'hard' liquors such as whisky and rum but rather the fermented varieties such as beer and wine. Although beer and wine have a lower percentage of alcohol than distilled spirits, fermented liquors retain all of the metabolic wastes produced by the yeast during the fermentation process – in effect 'yeast poop' – and these fermentive wastes are highly acid-forming and toxic to the tissues. The liver bears the major burden of processing all the acids and toxic wastes that enter the body and pollute the bloodstream whenever beer and wine are drunk and, if fermented liqours are consumed daily, the liver gradually succumbs to toxic overload, swelling up and hardening with residual toxic waste until cirrhosis develops. To make matters worse, most commercial beers and wines today contain chemical contaminants such as formaldehyde, preservatives, artificial dyes, flavouring agents and other toxic additives, all of which contribute more to blood acidosis, tissue toxicity and the gradual erosion of the liver. In terms of their effects on health and longevity, except for an occasional glass of an exceptionally good vintage or brew with dinner, beer and wine are not good choices as intoxicants for daily use, especially for 'social drinking', when one tends to drink to excess, because the 'cost/benefit' ratio is far too high.

Distilled spirits, which are refined from fermented liquors, are a much 'cleaner' form of alcohol for human consumption because the distillation process completely eliminates all the other toxic by-products of fermentation, leaving only pure distilled alcohol. While distilled spirits such as vodka and brandy have a higher alcohol content than beer or wine, they are usually consumed in much smaller amounts per drink than fermented beverages, and therefore they deliver the same basic dose of alcohol into the bloodstream.

Known for centuries in Western Europe as *eau de vie*, the 'water of life', and in ancient China as *jiou-jing*, the 'essence of wine', distilled spirits were originally used more for therapeutic, medicinal purposes than for recreational intoxication. Used properly and in moderation, spirits have potent medicinal properties that may be used to treat a variety of conditions, including sluggish circulation, insufficient body heat, low metabolic rate and nervous tension. The slightly intoxicating effect on the mind produced by small doses of spirits adds an extra dimension to its therapeutic applications, and this psycho-active influence is well reflected in the term chosen to denote distilled alcohol – spirits.

All distilled spirits, including brandy and whisky, are crystal clear and completely pure after the distillation process. The distinctive amber colour and characteristic flavour in various types of whisky, brandy and other tinted spirits come from the resins leached from the wooden casks in which these liquors are aged. This aging process leaves tannins and other toxic resins suspended in the spirits, and these must all be processed by the liver along with the toxic metabolites of alcohol itself. Therefore, the healthiest choice in spirits are the clear varieties that have not been aged in wooden casks, such as vodka, gin, tequila and white rum.

Throughout East Asia, people drink a type of medicinal spirit prepared by steeping potent tonic herbs in distilled spirits for three to six months, then straining the infused liquor into bottles and taking it in measured dosages on a daily basis, particularly in the winter. Known in China as *yao jiou* ('medicine liquor') or *chwun-jiou* ('spring wine'), this ancient herbal tonic has been used for thousands of years throughout the Far East as a means of preserving health, boosting vitality and prolonging life, as well as for its relaxing effects. The alcohol extracts and preserves all the essential active ingredients from the various tonic herbs, delivering them swiftly into the bloodstream directly through the stomach and providing a strong metabolic boost to the therapeutic potency of the herbal essences. Medicinal spirits are an excellent delivery system for the life-prolonging therapeutic benefits of herbal tonics such as ginseng, astragalus and wolf-berry, while also serving the 'recreational' function of liquor. This is a good example of how the 'art of rational retox' may be applied to transform a 'toxic intoxicant' into a 'tonic intoxicant', thereby reducing the costs to health and increasing the benefits to longevity of drinking alcohol. Readers who wish to add a therapeutic dimension to their recreational drinking will find the formula for preparing excellent traditional Chinese tonic spirits in the Recipes and Formulas section on page 335.

Tips for tipplers and smokers

If you drink and/or smoke daily, it's important to take a few basic precautions to counteract the additional acidity, toxicity and dehydration which alcohol and tobacco produce in the body. Alcohol in particular dehydrates the blood and tissues, and it's therefore necessary to drink a few extra glasses of alkaline water each day, both to flush out the toxic acid wastes and to rehy-drate the blood and cellular fluids. If the water you drink is charged with negative ions, it has even greater detoxifying and rehydrating activity in the tissues and helps protect the liver from damage by the toxic metabolites of alcohol and tobacco in the bloodstream.

People who smoke and drink regularly should also take extra rations of antioxidant nutrients, particularly vitamins E, C and betacarotene, plus a full spectrum mineral supplement to replace the essential minerals and trace elements depleted from the tissues by alcohol and tobacco. It's also a good idea to take some form of 'green food' supplement as a source of organic chloro-phyll and other cleansing elements to purify the blood and cellular fluids.

One of the most effective antidotes of all against the toxic damage caused by daily use of alcohol, tobacco and other intox-icants is to drink High Mountain Oolung Tea (*gao-shan oolung cha*), especially first thing in the morning and again late in the afternoon, which is how many smokers and drinkers in China, Taiwan and Japan protect their bodies from the hazards of their habits. Recent scientific research has confirmed the efficacy of High Mountain Oolung Tea as a potent blood purifier, tissue detoxificant, alkalizer and preventive against cancer. It is particularly effective in preventing toxic damage to the tissues of the lungs and the liver, which are precisely the organs that smokers and drinkers must take special measures to purify and protect. Here again we see how the 'art of rational retox' transforms an ordinary daily beverage such as tea into an extraordinary therapeutic drink that protects health and prolongs life.

CHAPTER 13

Advice on Medicinal and Recreational Drugs

In the previous chapter, we discussed the dubious distinction between 'therapeutic' and 'recreational' use of the legal drugs tobacco and alcohol, and we saw how so-called 'recreational drugs' can also have useful therapeutic applications. In this chapter, we'll expand the scope of this discussion to include all drugs – medicinal and recreational, chemical and herbal, synthetic and natural – and try to establish a few basic guidelines for a rational approach to using these substances.

To begin with, we must admit the fact that, just as many people smoke tobacco and drink alcohol more for therapeutic than recreational reasons, so a lot of people take medicinal drugs more for recreational than therapeutic purposes. It's hard to tell whether people who've been taking the same pharmaceutical drug every day for over ten years continue to use it because they still have the same therapeutic need for it as when the drug was first prescribed, or because they've grown fond of its effects and continue to take it simply because they like it, not because they need it.

The reason this point is so important is that many people assume that just because their doctors prescribe a particular drug for a particular condition at a particular time, that the drug must therefore be safe to take any time, or even all the time, with or

without the original condition. This is a false and often dangerous assumption: in America alone, more than 100,000 people die
each year as a direct result of using pharmaceutical drugs, and
several hundred thousand more are hospitalized each and every
year due to severe adverse reactions to these drugs. In the UK,
the pharmaceutical chain Boots was forced, in April 1993, to
reveal that its heart drug Manoplax could lead to higher mortality. Clinical trials showed that patients with severe congestive
heart failure taking 100 mg of Manoplax had 'significantly
increased risk of death compared with those not receiving the
drug'. The same point applies to people who rationalize their
heavy use of alcohol and tobacco by telling themselves it must
be safe because it's legal. In both cases, the consumer suffers
serious, sometimes fatal, harm as a result of ignorance regarding
the basic facts about the drugs they use, facts which their doctors
and commercial advertising usually fail to mention.

People who wish to preserve their health and prolong their
lives should exercise the same basic precautions when selecting
medicinal and recreational drugs as they do when selecting food.
Would you start eating a new food product and include it in
your daily diet without first finding out what's in it, simply
because the person who sells it assures you that it's good for
you? The same rule which governs choice in food applies to
drugs as well: if it's derived from natural plant, animal or mineral
sources, then it's acceptable; if it's synthesized from artificial
chemical sources, it should be rejected. This rule applies both to
medicinal and recreational drugs, for, as noted in the previous
chapter, it doesn't matter to the body whether a substance is
taken for therapy or for pleasure. Either way, it produces the
same physiological effects and psychological side effects in the
body and mind of the user.

The next time your doctor prescribes you a new pharmaceutical drug, ask him or her to tell you what the basic ingredients
are. Many doctors don't have a clue how to answer that question,

because they have nothing to do with the production of the drugs they prescribe. However, as a consumer it's your right to know what's in the drugs you are prescribed, and it's the doctor's duty to inform you. In TCM, doctors always tell their patients precisely what ingredients are used to prepare their herbal prescriptions, and how the herbs react with various foods and other medications, and patients can request that particular ingredients be deleted, added or substituted, based on their own personal requirements. If patients really knew what most modern pharmaceutical drugs are made of, many would be so revolted that they'd refuse to take them and switch to traditional medicine instead. Swallowing a pill on the word of a doctor who doesn't know what's in it, how it's made or how it reacts with other things is definitely not a rational way to take medicine.

The primary consideration when deciding what sorts of drugs to use, medicinally or recreationally, is to ensure that they come from natural organic sources and are free of toxic chemical additives. In traditional medicine such as TCM and ayurveda, medicinal drugs were always made from plants, minerals and animal parts, and those with intoxicating side effects, such as opium, cannabis, datura and numerous others, were not separated into a special class known as 'recreational drugs'. While it's certainly true that medicinal drugs with intoxicating properties were sometimes taken for recreational purposes, they still remained legitimate medicines with therapeutic properties, and their occasional recreational use was of no concern to anyone but the user. Since all herbal intoxicants are organic compounds from natural sources, their moderate use does not do serious harm to health, whether taken for medicinal or recreational reasons, and their metabolites are easily excreted from the body.

In the past, when a patient had a therapeutic need for a particular medicinal herb that happened to have intoxicating side effects, such as opium or hemp, the 'recreational' side effect became either a bonus or a nuisance to the patient, depending on his or her individual proclivities, but it never became a legal issue, as it has today. A good example of this is the smoking of cannabis hemp to control pain, restore appetite and assist digestion and assimilation in cancer and AIDS patients, all of whom testify that this herb is only effective for this purpose when the whole natural herb is smoked, and that the orally administered synthetic substitutes prescribed by doctors are totally useless. For these patients, the 'high' produced by smoking this herb is a mere side effect, enjoyed by some as a pleasant sensation and simply tolerated by others as an annoying distraction, but it's not their primary reason for using it. Indeed, doctors routinely give AIDS and cancer patients extremely toxic chemotherapy and other dangerous pharmaceutical drugs that have devastating side effects and may kill them, but that doesn't prevent them from continuing to prescribe these drugs, nor has it prompted their prohibition. However, when these same patients request a medicinal herb with proven efficacy for their conditions and a harmless intoxicating side effect, it's denied to them as a 'dangerous drug'. Small wonder that most people today are confused on this issue.

While traditional medicine still relies entirely on herbs and other natural products, modern allopathic medicine employs thousands of chemically synthesized drugs produced by the pharmaceutical industry and prescribed by doctors for virtually all ailments. Many of these drugs are made from highly toxic, often carcinogenic, chemicals, such as coal tar. Coal tar is a poisonous by-product of the petroleum industry and was originally disposed of as a hazardous waste, until chemists discovered that it could be used to synthesize a wide range of chemical drugs, including some with intoxicating properties, such as painkillers and sleeping pills. Many pharmaceutical drugs are made from inorganic substances that are extremely difficult to excrete from the body, and their toxic residues do untold damage to the liver and other tissues in which they accumulate. All chemical drugs cause highly acid-forming re-actions in the bloodstream and depress the body's internal self-cleansing and excretory functions, resulting in a state of severe toxaemia. Unless absolutely necessary for short-term therapy, synthetic pharmaceutical drugs should be strictly avoided, and natural herbal medicines used instead.

Precisely the same advice applies to the use of recreational drugs: if they come from natural sources and have not been contaminated with toxic chemicals, they are relatively 'user-friendly'; if they are made of synthetic substances, they are truly 'dangerous drugs'. Examples of the latter category are all amphetamines such as 'speed' (methamphetamine), 'ecstasy' and other 'uppers', all sleeping pills, sedatives, tranquillizers, and other 'downers', and all chemical narcotics, including heroin and cocaine. Even though heroin and cocaine are extracted from natural plant sources – opium and coca leaf respectively – there are so many industrial solvents and other toxic chemicals used in the refinement process that these two drugs are just as hazardous as synthetic narcotics. If you're in serious pain and need a natural narcotic painkiller, ask the doctor for morphine or codeine, both of which are organic alkaloids extracted from whole herbal opium and therefore compatible with human metabolism and easily excreted from the body.

Pharmaceutical drugs that are used for recreational purposes are the most dangerous of all because they are designed to directly stimulate or sedate the brain and central nervous system by over riding or by-passing natural neurological functions, and their toxic metabolites can do permanent damage to highly sensitive brain and nerve cells, while also causing serious behavioural and emotional disorders. These neuro-active chemical drugs are also very addictive. Because they're mostly inorganic, it's much more difficult to flush their toxic residues from the body than it is to eliminate the metabolites of natural organic compounds, which makes these addictions extremely difficult to break. Using such drugs is simply not worth the damage it does to the body, nor does it conform with the principles of 'rational retox'.

If, however, you have a condition that requires the use of a synthetic pharmaceutical drug, you should take similar protective measures as those suggested for daily use of tobacco and alcohol. Drink a few extra glasses each day of alkaline, preferably ionized, water to help flush out the toxic metabolites which these drugs leave in the blood and liver. Take some extra antioxidant supplements, such as vitamins C, E and betacarotene, as well as 'green food' to keep the bloodstream clean. When using chemically produced drugs, especially for prolonged periods, it's also a good idea to take liquid bentonite ('clay water') for a few days each week, or for a full week each month, to thoroughly purify the bloodstream and cleanse the cellular fluids of the residual acids and inorganic toxins which these drugs leave in the body. The negatively charged bentonite molecules saturate the bodily fluids and absorb the positively charged toxic particles like a vacuum cleaner sucking in dust from a carpet, and this helps prevent the cellular damage that invariably occurs if such toxins are permitted to accumulate for too long in the tissues.

Another factor that sometimes requires counterbalancing is the drastic drop in blood sugar which these drugs often cause, especially those which directly influence the central nervous system and have intoxicant properties. Such drugs significantly increase metabolic activity in the brain and nerve cells, greatly increasing their demand for glucose, which is the only fuel that brain and nerve tissue can utilize. Consequently, these drugs cause the brain and nerves to drain the bloodstream of all available supplies of glucose, depleting reserves and causing a sharp, swift drop in blood sugar levels. This in turn causes dizziness and lethargy, weakness and confusion, chills and palpitations, and other unpleasant symptoms of hypoglycaemia; it often triggers anxiety attacks as well.

The best way to offset this effect is to quickly replenish the bloodstream's supply of glucose by eating something that contains a concentrated natural sweetener, such as honey, maple syrup or raw cane sugar, or else some sweet ripe fruit, such as banana, papaya or peach. Best of all is to eat fresh black grapes, or drink freshly extracted grape juice, which contains abundant supplies of natural glucose, or 'blood sugar'. Unlike fructose and other complex sugars in most fruits and natural sweeteners, glucose does not require conversion in the body in order to become bio-available as fuel for the brain and nerves. The glucose in grapes is assimilated directly into the bloodstream from the stomach, providing swift relief from the symptoms of low blood sugar, and refueling the brain and nerves with fresh supplies of glucose. Black grapes also contain elements which detoxify the blood and liver, protecting the body against damage from the toxic metabolites produced by chemical drugs. Eating fresh black grapes is therefore a quick remedy for the 'sugar blues' of hypoglycaemia, and a good way to take the raw edge off harsh pharmaceutical drugs.

CHAPTER 14

Setting Your Detox/Retox Clocks

A key strategy for protecting health, preventing disease and prolonging life is to align your personal lifestyle with the natural patterns of your body's basic biorhythms, and to regulate your daily habits in ways that set your body's internal 'detox/retox clocks' to activate periodic cycles of internal cleansing and healing responses. Detox/retox is a cyclical process: blood and tissue toxicity gradually increases until it reaches the critical stage, at which point the body's built-in detox mechanisms are activated and quickly remove the offending toxins, thereby restoring the original state of purity and functional balance, after which another retox cycle begins, and so forth. This is a physiological manifestation of the primordial interplay of yin and yang within the body, the same polar principle that runs throughout all dimensions of nature and operates within the body in overlapping cycles of time – daily, weekly, monthly and yearly (Fig. 12).

When allowed to function naturally, without human artifice or external interference, the body's self-toxifying (retox) and self-detoxifying (detox) cycles operate smoothly and efficiently, maintaining a homeostatic state of balance that supports health and prolongs life. However, for every artificial factor that we add to nature's carefully balanced equations of life – such as

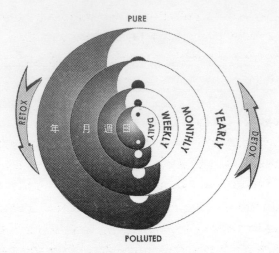

Fig. 12 **Natural detox/retox cycles and the 'wheels of time'**

denatured diets, chemical drugs, electromagnetic and microwave pollution, contaminated air and water – we must take specific counteractive measures to compensate for the imbalances and correct the deviations which these factors produce in our internal detox/retox cycles. The most effective way to restore your body's natural detox/retox rhythms is to adapt your personal lifestyle to allow the body's internal self-cleansing mechanisms to catch up with the toxic overload on a daily, weekly, monthly and yearly basis.

Let's briefly recall the analogy of maintaining a car, with which we launched this discussion in the Preface. Just as a car needs to have its motor tuned, its internal parts cleaned and its oil and other fluids replenished on a regular basis in order to perform properly, avoid breakdowns, and prolong its 'mileage life', so the human body requires regular maintenance and internal cleansing in order to stay healthy, prevent disease and prolong life. And like a car, as well as major annual maintenance and repair programmes, the human body must also be fed the right fuel and properly cared for on a day-to-day basis in order to prevent excessive wear and tear and reduce production of toxic wastes. And in addition to annual and daily maintenance, there are also some things that may be done on a weekly and monthly basis to improve the body's performance and reduce its rate of deterioration.

Yearly maintenance

The seven-day detox and internal cleansing fast with colonic irrigation, as discussed in Chapter 6, is the best way to periodically detoxify the blood and tissues, rebalance the body and regenerate vital functions on a yearly basis. It's also one of the most effective ways to prolong life. This programme removes the hard, deeply impacted mucus and putrefactive wastes which accumulate in the wall of the bowels, thereby eliminating the main source of blood and tissue toxicity in the body. Since these toxic wastes are a major cause of tissue degeneration, organ failure, fatigue and other symptoms of ageing, totally eliminating them from the body once a year with a seven-day fast and colonic irrigations is the best way to slow down the ageing process and extend human lifespan. Exactly seven days of fasting are required for this detox cycle to completely purify the bloodstream and detoxify the tissues and cellular fluids, and if you do this regularly, once a year, all sorts of diseases and degenerative conditions are nipped in the bud and never have a chance to develop.

A yearly one-week cleansing fast may also serve as an annual withdrawal programme to gradually give up old food addictions and break bad eating habits. Each time you do this programme, it becomes progressively easier to adopt wholesome new food choices and cultivate better eating habits. This annual 'house cleaning' allows you to indulge in a bit of overeating, drinking and other bingeing during the course of the year, then clears your body of all the residual toxic debris in one clean sweep, before it can do any serious damage.

Another yearly maintenance programme that promotes

health and longevity is to take all or part of your annual holiday in the form of a 'health holiday' at your favourite resort, beach or mountain retreat. This new style of vacation is becoming quite popular, and there are now many spas and health resorts that provide packaged health holiday programmes that include various detox and healing therapies. Rather than exhaust your energy and pollute your body with all the hectic activity and overindulgence that characterizes conventional holiday plans, try giving your body and mind a *real* vacation from the stress and strain of daily life by resting quietly at a cosy spa, a deluxe beach resort or a simple mountain cabin, eating only fresh, lightly cooked vegetarian food, drinking only pure alkaline water, pampering your tired, toxic body with heliotherapy, herbal steam, hot mineral baths, massage, or just snoozing in a hammock. The money you save by not eating at expensive restaurants, not dancing in fancy nightclubs, not shopping and not spending on the other extravagances of conventional holidays can be used instead to pay for pure, simple foods and basic therapeutic services that cleanse and repair the body rather than pollute and damage it. Instead of returning to work tired and hung-over from non-stop partying, you'll resume your daily routines with renewed vitality and fully replenished resources. If you like to party, it's best to do it on weekends, one party at a time, and give yourself a full day to recover afterwards. Long holidays, however, are more wisely used for real rest and relaxation.

Monthly maintenance

A traditional Asian regimen for monthly maintenance of the body is to ingest only water and fresh fruit juice for three days each month, starting on the day of the new moon in order to time the internal cleansing and regeneration process with the beginning of a new lunar cycle. To further increase the detox benefits of this regimen, you may also take a dose or two of ground psyllium seed shaken in water on each of these three days. This clears the bowels of putrid digestive debris and makes you feel less hungry owing to the bulking properties of psyllium. This is also a good time to do daily sessions with the Zapper (see page 232) in order to eliminate parasites from the body along with all the other toxic wastes.

Some people, especially heavy meat-eaters, cannot go for three days each month on nothing but fruit and water without triggering a major detox reaction that interferes with work and other daily activities. In that case, a less rigorous monthly maintenance programme is to take one full week each month eating only a purely vegetarian diet, without any meat, eggs or dairy products. While this is not as detoxifying as a three-day fruit and water programme, it does effectively counteract acidosis in the blood and tissues, which is the biggest health problem caused by eating animal products. For someone accustomed to eating meat, eggs and dairy products every day, eating only fresh vegetables, fruit and whole grains for seven days each month serves as a sort of semi-fast, but without the intensive detox reactions and 'healing crisis' of a real fast. This is also a very good way for meat-eaters to discover how much better they feel when they cut down on animal products in their diets, and to gradually work their way towards trying a genuine therapeutic cleansing fast – first for only one day, then for three days, and finally for seven days.

Weekly maintenance

An alternative way to allow your body to detoxify and rebalance itself on a regular basis is to spend one day each week consuming nothing but water and fresh fruit. This gives the bowels a chance to catch up with the backlog of waste elimination, rebalances the digestive organs and restores proper pH in the blood and tissues. Since no cooked food is consumed on that day, the enzymes normally used for digestive purposes are diverted to assist tissue cleansing and immune functions instead.

The cleansing and healing benefits of this weekly day of digestive rest may be further enhanced by soaking in a hot bath with
Epsom or Celtic sea salts and a dash of detoxifying essential oils,
such as grapefruit, rosemary or sage. Deep-tissue massage,
herbal steam and infrared sauna are other good ways to amplify
the cleansing and rebalancing benefits of a weekly day of rest
and relaxation. In fact, simply by remaining at rest for 24 hours
and abstaining from cooked food you permit your body to shift
into the healing mode of the parasympathetic branch of the
nervous system, and this brief respite from the stress and strain
of daily life suffices to recharge and rebalance the body and
repair minor damage to tissues caused by weekly wear and tear.
If you do this every week, that amounts to 52 days a year of rest
rather than stress, waste elimination rather than waste accumulation, regeneration instead of degeneration. The cumulative
benefits to health and longevity of such a weekly programme
are almost as great as a monthly three-day fast on fruit and
water, and it's a good alternative for those who'd rather not
spend three days in a row each month without eating solid food.

Daily maintenance
The best way to support health and longevity on a day-to-day
basis is to enlist the elements of air and water to assist daily
detox and help keep the bloodstream properly balanced. First
thing each morning, before eating any food, drink two glasses
of ionized, alkaline micro-clustered water to flush mucus and
acids from the stomach, give the bloodstream an alkaline boost
and rehydrate the cells and tissues. This infusion of energized
alkaline water establishes proper pH balance in all the blood
and other vital fluids of the body and boosts cellular metabolism with the ionized alkaline minerals required for optimum
energy production. By starting each day this way, you flush out
residual acids and toxins from the previous day and replenish

your blood and tissues with pure, properly balanced water, establishing the conditions for optimum metabolic efficiency throughout the day.

The air element may be harnessed by practising 15–20 minutes of *tu-na* or other *chi gung* breathing exercises immediately after drinking those two glasses of water and before eating breakfast. Deep breathing exercises practised early in the morning expel residual carbon dioxide and other gaseous wastes from the bloodstream, replenishing the blood and cellular fluids with abundant supplies of fresh oxygen and negative ion energy. Deep diaphragmatic breathing also alkalizes the bloodstream, and helps establish proper pH balance throughout the body. Two glasses of pure alkaline water followed by 20 minutes of deep breathing is the true 'breakfast of champions', and this simple morning regimen will not only add more years to your life, but also add more life to your years.

In addition to starting each day with an alkaline and oxygen boost from air and water, proper daily health care requires that the diet be regulated according the basic rules of food combining, and complemented with a few special supplements to facilitate internal cleansing and provide complete nutritional balance. Herbal detox teas, 'green foods', digestive enzymes and various full-spectrum vitamin and mineral supplements may all be judiciously used to help keep the body balanced and properly nourished on a daily basis. By eating food in a way that delivers optimum nutrition with minimum production of toxic waste, the body's daily elimination and self-cleansing cycles don't get overloaded and tissue toxicity never builds up to damaging levels. The lower you keep the level of toxicity in your body, the longer you extend the duration of your life.

CHAPTER 15

'Don't Worry, Be Happy, Feel Good'

These six words are printed across the top of the calling card of actor Larry Hagman, who portrayed the nefarious, pugnacious character 'JR' in the popular television series *Dallas*. After spending 50 years of his life drinking champagne and orange juice for breakfast and lunch, then continuing throughout the afternoon and evening with vodka and orange juice, Hagman finally burned out his liver, which collapsed and ceased functioning as a result of chronic alcohol toxicity. His only hope of survival was to have a complete liver transplant, an operation with statistically slim chances of success, especially for a life-long alcoholic in his late sixties.

Nevertheless, Hagman survived the ordeal, and today he still flashes that winning roguish grin which made 'JR' famous. Having restored his vitality and reformed his lifestyle, Hagman continues to enjoy his new way of life as much as he did his old ways. By applying his 'Don't worry, be happy, feel good' philosophy as much to his present 'therapeutic' recovery stage as he did to his former 'recreational' drinking days, Hagman has managed to survive the hazards of both and enjoy one as much as the other. As Norman Cousins, another man who laughed his way to a complete recovery from a supposedly 'incurable' disease, wrote in his memoirs, 'The will to live is not a theoretical abstraction, but a physiologic reality with therapeutic characteristics.' So potent is the 'power of positive thinking' that it can stimulate the body to cure itself of conditions that modern medicine regards as irreparable and fatal.

The 'JR attitude' of carefree, happy-go-lucky hedonism reflected in Hagman's motto is a lot more than just a cheerful slogan. When you 'don't worry', your ardenal glands don't secrete stress hormones such as cortisone, which suppress immune response and enervate the nervous system with hypertension. When you are 'happy', your brain secretes neuropeptides, the 'happy hormones' that communicate directly with the glands of the endocrine system and signal them to 'turn on the juice' of healing hormones and other immune factors. The invariable result of this biofeedback between the neuropeptides produced by a happy mind and the healing hormones required for a healthy body is that you 'feel good' both in body and in mind. This balanced state of health and happiness is sustained by specific neuropathways and endocrine channels through which these secretions communicate in every part of the body.

While the right attitude is without doubt the most fundamental factor in health, as it is in all aspects of living, there are some things in life that require technique and discipline as well, and detox is one of the most important of these. Detox is no tea party. It's a tiresome, sometimes gruelling experience, especially if you're highly toxic when you start. As the internal cleansing process moves progressively into deeper layers of tissue and releases more and more toxic residues into the bloodstream for excretion, all sorts of unpleasant detox symptoms can manifest themselves, including headache and body pain, insomnia and fatigue, fever and chills, irritability and anger. It's reassuring to know that the worse you feel during detox, the better the programme is working for you and the more toxins you're draining out of your body, but you still have to endure the process. It's also rewarding to realize that the cumulative toxicity from years of indiscriminate eating, drinking and other careless habits can be completely flushed out of the body and much of the damage repaired with just a week or two of an intensive, disciplined detox programme. Of course, this, too, requires more than just the right techniques – it also requires the right attitude. And it calls for time, patience and a period of real rest and relaxation.

Activating the complementary relationship between a happy mind and a healthy body is one of the great achievements made possible by the power of positive thinking. Today, the neuro-immunological link between a positive state of mind and a positive state of health has become known in modern medicine as psychoneuroimmunology, or PNI, but in traditional holistic medicine it's been recognized as a basic fact of life for thousands of years. The 2,000-year-old Chinese medical text known as the *Internal Medicine Classic* states, 'If one maintains an undisturbed spirit within, no disease will occur.' In *Maximum Immunity*, Dr Michael Weiner echoes the same premise in more technical terms when he writes, 'By learning how to control our mind, subtle hormonal changes emerge that control our biochemical reality.'

Among the subtle hormonal changes stimulated in the body by the mind is the so-called 'placebo effect', whereby a patient who's given a sugar pill, but is told that he's taking a marvellous new medicine that will cure his disease, becomes so hopeful and happy that his mind triggers his own internal healing responses and he completely recovers. The placebo effect is produced entirely by the healing biofeedback between 'happy neuropeptides' from the brain and 'healthy hormones' in the endocrine system, and in many double-blind clinical trials to test new drugs, the placebo cures the patient just as often as the drug itself. Pharmaceutical companies regard this all-too-human healing response as an unfortunate nuisance, and are quick to discount it as an insignificant quirk, but in fact a positive outlook is the first and most important step in curing any ailment, and the main 'active ingredient' comes from the mind, not from a pill.

The corollary principle to the power of positive thinking is the power of pessimism and negative emotion, which is every bit as destructive to health and longevity as a positive attitude is constructive. Stress and all the negativity it engenders in the mind have become primary causes of disease and degenerative conditions throughout the Western world, as well as in many newly developed Asian societies. Cortisone and other stress hormones set the stage for heart disease, cancer, stroke, hypertension, chronic infections, ulcers, immune deficiency and many other crippling conditions. Stress factors such as cortisone have also been linked to high rates of suicide in modern industrialized countries. As Dr Weiner points out in *Maximum Immunity*, 'Psychological stress releases powerful hormones that suppress our immune defences.' In *Eat Right or Die Young*, Dr Cass Igram cites stress and negative emotions as the main causes of cancer and immune deficiency:

> The role played by stress in the causation of cancer is so great that it would not be an exaggeration to say that 80 per cent or more cancer cases have their immediate origin in some form of mental pressure or strain. Grief, distress, fear, worry and anger are emotions which have horrible effects on the body's functions. Researchers have discovered that these emotions cause the release of chemicals from the brain . . . [that] have a profound immune-suppressive action. Scientists have traced a pathway from the brain to the immune cells proving that negative emotions can stop the immune cells dead in their tracks.

Just as the powers of positive and negative thinking have decisive effects on human health and longevity, so the 'power of proper pH′ has a strong influence on balance in body and mind. Alkaline blood and cellular fluids support a healthy body and promote a happy mind, while blood and tissue acidosis paves the way for disease and decay and gives rise to depression, tension, anger, fear and other negative mental and emotional states. A good example of this is the extreme state of acidosis suffered by many children today due to excessive consumption of refined sugar, starch and dairy products: not only does this sort of diet cause diabetes, obesity, tooth decay and other physical defects, the high acidity it produces in the blood and tissues is also a major factor in hyperactivity, attention deficit disorder, violence, depression, suicide and other debilitating behavioural disorders. Doctors in America have responded to this growing blight of childhood malaise by giving these children powerful amphetamines and anti-depressants to suppress their symptoms, but this chemical drug therapy only further aggravates the root cause of the problem and does nothing to cure it. Usually in such cases, a thorough detox and a complete re-alkalization of the blood and tissues, followed by strict dietary reform, are all that's needed to correct both the physical and the mental and emotional disorders caused by chronic acidosis in children as well as adults. In order for any real healing to occur, the state of the body and the state of the mind must be considered as two sides of the same coin and treated as inseparably linked aspects of the same conditions.

Almost everyone likes to 'eat, drink, and be merry', but few of us wish to die 'tomorrow'. The human body is a complex engine that serves both as a workhorse and as a vehicle for enjoying life's pleasures. It's therefore important to learn how to operate and maintain the body properly, so that it doesn't break down in the middle of life's journey and leave you stranded in a wheelchair or sickbed. The human body is genetically designed to last for about 120 years, and barring accidents and other unforeseen events, it can remain fully functional for the full term of its natural 120-year lifespan – as long as it's properly cared for along the way. There's no point in living long unless you are able to remain active and continue enjoying life until the end, and that requires careful attention to the basic facts and functions of life.

One of the most important factors, and the one upon which everything else depends, is the right attitude, without which health cannot be maintained and healing cannot be achieved. Patients who have an attitude problem, whether it be cynical, resentful, angry, paranoid, pessimistic or any other form of psycho-emotional 'dis-ease', must first purify their thoughts and detoxify their emotions before they can benefit from any sort of physical cleansing therapies. Negative emotional and mental states not only block the body's detox and healing responses, they also produce a constant stream of toxic metabolites and acid-forming reactions, thereby negating the positive benefits of any healing therapy.

The human experience suggests that positive mental factors such as joy, love and hope are even more decisive than therapeutic physical factors such as diet, herbs and exercise in determining the state of human health and the length of human life. People who know how to relax and enjoy life, and who take 'Don't worry, be happy, feel good' as their guiding motto, often live longer, healthier lives – even while eating, drinking and living precisely as they please – than those who constantly worry about their health and dread death. With the right attitude, you can push your body to amazing limits in the pursuit of fortune and pleasure, then pull back from the brink of disaster and repair the damage just in the nick of time to enjoy your sunset years as well. And if you still have any doubts about the power of 'attitude' to renew a life nearly lost, go ask 'JR' to explain the meaning of 'Don't worry, be happy, feel good!'

Recipes and Formulas

Thai herbal steam formulas

Any steambath may be turned into an herbal steam simply by adding the appropriate herbs directly to the water in the boiler. The active herbal essences vaporize along with the steam from the water and enter the steam chamber along with the steam. When using fresh herbs, a total of about 400 g of the chopped herbs is sufficient for a small steamroom; when the herbs are in dried form, use about half that amount. Fresh and dried herbs may also be used together. Precise proportions are not important, but generally you may use equal quantities of each herb, adding more or less of the ones which you personally prefer. Three popular formulas are given below, but feel free to experiment with other combinations and different aromatic herbs.

Basic Thai herbal steam formula

lemongrass (preferably fresh)   galanga root ('Thai ginger')
wild lime   black peppercorn
ginger   morning glory (preferably fresh)
sage

Formula for arthritis and inflammation

lemongrass (preferably fresh)	galanga root ('Thai ginger')
wild lime	greenbriar
ginger	rosemary
sage	cinnamon

Formula to assist sleep and relaxation

lemongrass (preferably fresh)	lavender
ginger	mandarin orange
sage	thyme
jasmine	

Clear vegetable broth for detox diet

2 litres pure water
1 tsp Celtic sea salt
5 slices ginger root
2 carrots, finely chopped
3 stalks celery, finely chopped
115 g cabbage, finely chopped
175 g spinach, finely chopped
225 g pumpkin, finely diced
1 squash, finely chopped
5 shitake mushrooms (fresh or dried), finely sliced
1 bunch parsley, chopped

Place all the ingredients in a large, non-aluminium cooking pot. Bring to a full boil, then reduce the heat to a simmer, cover partially with a lid, and let it cook until the liquid is reduced to about half. Line a colander with a piece of muslin cloth, and strain the broth into a bowl. Discard the vegetable pulp, and drink the broth with meals or as a snack between meals.

Job's Tears and brown rice porridge

Herbal porridges have been part of the Chinese diet since ancient times, serving the dual functions of food and medicine. They are very easy to prepare and lend themselves to infinite variations in flavour and therapeutic effects. The recipe below is one of the oldest on record and combines the balanced nutrition of brown rice with the decongestant, anti-inflammatory and cooling therapeutic effects of Job's Tears (*Coix lacryma-jobi*). A few additional variations are given at the end of the recipe.

Wash and rinse 225 g brown rice together with 85 g Job's Tears, then place in a large, non-aluminium cooking pot with 2.5 litres of pure water and set aside to soak for 3–4 hours, or overnight. When ready to cook, add 1 teaspoon Celtic sea salt, bring to a full boil, cover with a lid, and lower the heat to a simmer. Let it cook for about 1 ¼ hours, until the grain is soft and the liquid begins to thicken.

For savoury porridge, add ½ tsp Celtic sea salt, 1 teaspoon Chinese sesame oil and 1 tablespoon chopped spring onion to individual serving bowls, then fill the bowls with hot porridge and stir to blend.

For sweet porridge, add your choice of sweeteners such as maple syrup, raw sugar, honey, chopped dates, raisins or banana to individual serving bowls, then fill with hot porridge and stir to blend.

Variations

1) Add 75 g of dried lotus seeds to the rice and Job's Tears, plus an additional 250 ml of water to the cooking liquid. Lotus seeds add cardiotonic and nervine properties to the porridge, and also function as a sexual tonic.

2) Add 8–10 Chinese jujubes ('red dates') to the pot when cooking. These add both nutritional and tonic value to the porridge,

and are known in China for their long-term benefits to health and longevity.

3) For a richer flavour, better texture and extra nutritional value, try using 115 g wild rice and 115 g brown rice, rather than just brown rice.

4) If you're not vegetarian, you may substitute a rich chicken broth for the water when cooking the porridge, but be very sure to use only broth prepared from organically raised chickens. This increases the tonic properties of the porridge, and provides extra warming effects in cold weather.

Sage tea

According to Dr Rudolph Breuss, sage tea is the single most effective herbal tea for detoxifying the body and strengthening immunity and resistance on a daily basis. He recommends preparing a batch of sage tea first thing each morning, and drinking it throughout the day, every day, for life. His recipe for one day's dosage for one person is given below.

Bring 500 ml of pure water to the boil in a non-aluminium pot, lower the heat, and add 1 teaspoon of dried sage. Allow to simmer for precisely 3 minutes, then remove from heat, add ½ teaspoon St John's Wort and ½ teaspoon peppermint, cover with a lid, and let steep for exactly 10 minutes. Strain the tea into a vacuum flask or bottle, and discard the dregs. Drink about 100 ml 3–4 times daily, on an empty stomach.

Lemon flax shake

Grind 2 heaped tablespoons (about 30 g) of whole flaxseed in a coffee grinder or food processor, then place into a blender with 3–4 ice cubes and 250 ml of water. Add the juice of 1 whole lemon, and blend until smooth. Pour into a glass and drink slowly on an empty stomach. For extra liver detoxifying properties, add 1 tablespoon of ground milk thistle seed to the blend.

Rejuvelac

Drinking cabbage rejuvelac is an excellent way to replenish the 'friendly flora' of beneficial lactobacteria in the digestive tract. It may be used to restore healthy lactobacteria colonies in the bowels after therapeutic fasts, colonic irrigations, antibiotic therapy or long periods of poor dietary habits. It may also be used to stimulate sluggish digestion and improve lower bowel functions, and as a remedy for chronic constipation. For best results, use continuously for 30–45 days, and repeat at least once a year.

The first batch of rejuvelac should be prepared in the morning by placing 400 ml of pure water and 350 g of coarsely chopped fresh cabbage in a blender, and blending them together for just 30 seconds. If you don't have a blender, simply chop the cabbage finely with a knife and mix with the water.

Pour the mixture of cabbage and water into a large jar, cover loosely, and let it stand at room temperature for exactly three days. Then strain off the liquid and discard the cabbage dregs.

Immediately prepare your next batch by blending another 350 g chopped cabbage with 350 ml of pure water, then add 60 ml of the freshly made rejuvelac as a 'starter'. Pour this mixture into a clean jar, cover loosely, and let stand for just 24 hours to ferment. Repeat this process each morning to prepare the following day's batch of rejuvelac, using 60 ml of each day's batch as a fermentive starter for the next batch.

Store the remaining fermented rejuvelac in the refrigerator and take 100 ml three times per day, with meals. If you don't finish the batch by the end of the day, discard what remains, and use the fresh batch of rejuvelac the following day.

Good rejuvelac should have a slightly sour taste, like yoghurt, and is sometimes slightly fizzy, like mineral water. If the first batch smells putrid and has a slimy texture, discard it and start over. Once you get a good batch going, it replicates itself easily and may be continued indefinitely, as long as you prepare it daily. And remember: the first batch takes three full days to ferment, while all subsequent batches take only 24 hours.

Liver detox tea

This tea may be used to decongest and detoxify the liver and improve the circulation of blood and energy through liver tissues.

10 g dandelion root	10 g burdock root
2 g mugwort	5 g ginger
5 g fennel	5 g milk thistle

Mix the dried herbs with 1.5 litres of pure water and bring to the boil in a non-aluminium cooking pot. Simmer slowly for about 20 minutes, then remove from the heat and let stand for 10 minutes. Strain into a bottle and take 60–100 ml warm tea three times per day. Start at the lower dosage and gradually work up to higher doses. Extra tea may be kept fresh in the refrigerator, but each dose should be warmed before drinking.

Liver detox formula for alcohol and drug poisoning

This is a classical Chinese liver cleansing formula that has been specially adapted to deal with severe toxicity of the liver due to poisoning from excessive long-term use of alcohol and/or drugs. Known as 'Major Bupleurum with Artemisia Decoction', this is a very strong liver detox formula that must be used with considerable care. It has strong purgative properties for both the liver and the bowels, and it often prompts voluminous fluid bowel movements containing yellow-orange bile drained from the liver and gall bladder. It's very important to remain completely at rest while taking this formula, avoiding all excitement and stress, and to eat properly. During the course of treatment (7–14 days), do not eat any refined sugars and starches, avoid chilli and other stimulating spices, and eliminate chicken, eggs, red meat, dairy products and deep-fried foods from your diet. Eat only fresh vegetables, whole grains and fruit, or select one of the detox diets given in Chapter 5.

The proportions given below are for one day's dosage for one person. When ordering the formula in a Chinese herb shop, ask the assistant to mix individual one-day dosages and wrap each one in separate packets. A ten-day course of treatment would therefore require ten one-day packets of the mixed herbs, each containing the amounts given below.

Bupleurum falcatum (hare's ear)	6 g
Artemisia cappilaris	4 g
Pinellia temata	4 g
Zingiber officinale (ginger, fresh)	4 g
Scutellaria macrantha	3 g
Paeonia lactiflora (white peony)	3 g
Ziziphus vulgaris (Chinese jujube)	3 g
Gardenia florida	3 g
Poncirus trifoliata (trifoliate orange)	2 g
Rheum officinale (rhubarb)	2 g

Place all the ingredients in a clay Chinese herb cooking pot, or use a heatproof glass vessel, but do not use a metal pot. Add 900 ml pure water. Bring to a full boil, then lower the heat, cover with a lid, and let simmer slowly until the liquid is reduced by about half. Strain into a bottle or bowl, and discard the dregs. Divide into three equal doses and take one dose three times a day, on an empty stomach. Continue for 7–14 days.

Lymphatic detox tea

This herbal tea may be used during a short fast, or in conjunction with a detox diet, to specifically detoxify the lymphatic system. The proportions given below are sufficient to make enough tea for about three days. Keep the tea stored in the refrigerator, but be sure to warm each dose before drinking.

red root	2 g
red clover	5 g
echinacea root	3 g
lemon peel	5 g
ginger	2 g

Place all the ingredients in a non-aluminium pot, add 1 litre pure water, bring to a full boil, then lower the heat, cover, and simmer for 20 minutes. Strain the tea into a bottle, and drink 100 ml twice daily, on an empty stomach. A small amount of honey may be added for taste, if desired.

Breuss kidney tea

This is an excellent way to cleanse the kidneys and bladder, especially during a detox programme, when these excretory organs must work overtime to remove toxic wastes from the bloodstream; 100 ml of the tea should be taken three times daily, continuously for up to three weeks, but no longer than that. For a complete kidney cleanse, it's best to do the full three weeks, and to follow a detox diet at the same time. The amounts given below are sufficient for one person for three full weeks, but each day's dosage should be prepared fresh each morning.

horsetail	15 g
stinging nettle	10 g

| knotgrass | 8 g |
| St John's wort | 6 g |

Mix the chopped dried herbs together until they are well blended, and keep in a clean, well sealed jar.

To prepare one day's dosage, steep one pinch (the amount held between the thumb and first two fingers) in 250 ml boiling hot water for 10 minutes, then strain off the tea and set aside. Put the dregs into a non-aluminium pot, add 350 ml pure water, bring to the boil, then lower the heat and let simmer for 10 minutes. Strain off the tea, discard the dregs, and mix with the first cup. Drink 100 ml first thing in the morning, another 100 ml before lunch, and 100 ml at bedtime. Discard any leftover tea, and prepare a fresh batch the following day.

Bladder and urinary tract cleansing tea

This blend promotes the elimination of wastes through the kidneys, urinary tract and bladder, and cleanses the tissues of these organs. It's particularly useful for flushing residual toxins and acids out of the bladder and urinary tract during an internal cleansing programme, or after a period of excessive eating and drinking. It may be used in conjunction with therapeutic fasts and detox diets, or as a quick urinary system cleanser in the course of daily life.

yarrow	6 g
elderflowers	6 g
cleavers	6 g
dandelion leaf	6 g
sarsaparilla	6 g
peppermint	6 g

Place all the ingredients except the peppermint in a non-aluminium pot, add 1.5 litres of pure water, bring to a full boil, lower the heat and simmer for 10 minutes. Remove from the heat, add the peppermint, and let steep for a further 10 minutes. Strain into jars and keep refrigerated. Drink 100 ml, warm or cold, three times a day, on empty stomach. After one week, the dosage may be increased to 250 ml three times daily.

Chinese herbal constipation formula

Known as 'moisten bowel decoction', this formula was first recorded in a Chinese medical text in the year 1249 AD. It is designed to remedy chronic constipation caused by dry bowels, insufficient secretion of bodily fluids and blood deficiency, all of which are common conditions today, especially among the elderly and postpartum women. This formula lubricates the bowels and helps clear blockages in the intestinal tract, thereby facilitating regular bowel movements.

hemp seeds, roasted (*cannabis*)	5 g
peach kernels	5 g
rhubarb (*Rheum officinale*)	3 g
Angelica sinensis	3 g
Angelica pubescens (purple)	3 g

Place all the ingredients in a clay Chinese herb cooker or heat-proof glass pot (not a metal one), and add 350 ml pure water. Bring to a full boil, lower the heat, cover with a lid, and simmer until the liquid has been reduced by about half. Strain the liquid into a bowl, add a further 250 ml of water to the dregs, boil and simmer these again until reduced by half, then strain again. Combine the two strained liquids, and divide into three equal doses. Take one dose three times daily, on empty stomach, for one week, or until normal bowel movements are restored.

Carminative herbal tea for gas and flatulence

This tea may be taken daily as often as needed to help control gas and flatulence. To increase its carminative (gas-expelling) properties, you may add two or three drops of pure peppermint oil to each cup that is drunk.

peppermint	8 g
ginger	5 g
fennel	5 g
lemon peel	3 g
cardamon	3 g
liquorice	3 g

Place all the ingredients in a non-aluminium pot, add 1.5 litres pure water, bring to a full boil, then reduce the heat, cover with a lid, and simmer for 20 minutes. Remove from the heat and let steep for a further 10 minutes, then strain. Drink as required throughout the day. Store any extra tea in the refrigerator.

Nervine tea

This relaxing herbal tea may be used to counteract insomnia and irritability during an intensive detox programme, or in the course of daily life to relieve anxiety and nervous tension, and to promote sound sleep at night. It may be used daily for long periods without any negative side effects.

chamomile	6 g
lavender	6 g
passionflower	6 g
hops	4 g
catnip	4 g
St John's wort	4 g

Place all the ingredients into a non-aluminium pot, and 1.5 litres pure water, bring to a full boil, reduce the heat, cover with a lid, and let simmer for 10 minutes. Remove from the heat and let steep for a further 10 minutes. Strain the tea and discard the dregs. Drink 100 ml of the warm tea, 2–3 times daily, or as often as required. Store extra tea in the refrigerator, and warm each dose before drinking.

Tonic herbal spirits, or 'spring wine'

This formula for tonic herbal spirits is one of the most ancient on record in Chinese medical texts. Known as 'The Duke of Chou's Centenarian Liquor', it is said to have been the personal elixir of the great Duke of Chou, who founded China's ancient Chou Dynasty in the year 1123 BC. Its potent tonic properties increase semen production in men and stimulate hormone production in women. It also enhances immune response, stimulates circulation of blood and energy, and strengthens the kidneys and adrenal glands. Its benefits to health are cumulative over time, and long-term use builds strong immunity, raises resistance to disease and paves the path to longevity.

Polygonatum cirrhifolium	60 g
Astragalus hoantchy (astragalus)	60 g
Rhemannia glutinosa	36 g
Porio cocus (tuchahoe)	60 g
Cinnamomum cassia (cinnamon)	18 g
Angelica sinensis	36 g
Codonopsis dangshen	30 g
Liriope spicata (creeping lilyturf)	30 g
Atractylodes macrocephala	30 g
Lycium chinese (Chinese wolfberry)	30 g
Citrus reticulata	30 g

Comus officinalis (dogwood tree)	30 g
Ligusticum wallichii	30 g
Ledebouriella seseloides	30 g
Chinemys reevesii	30 g
Schisandra chinensis (schisandra)	24 g
Angelica pubescens (purple)	24 g

Place all the ingredients in a large glass or ceramic vessel of at least 8-litre capacity. Add 7 litres of vodka, rum or brandy, and seal the vessel so that it is air-tight. Set aside to steep for 36 days, giving the vessel a good shake once in a while to mix the ingredients. After 36 days, strain off half the liquor into clean glass bottles, then add three fresh bottles of spirits to the remaining brew. Seal again, set aside to steep for another 15 days, then strain off the entire batch into clean bottles and discard the used herbs. Add a few lumps of rock crystal sugar, or a few tablespoons of honey, to each bottle to balance the flavour and smooth the texture, then seal with cork or cap. The herbal spirits may be stored indefinitely without losing therapeutic potency.

Take 45 ml once a day in summer, or twice a day in winter, on an empty stomach. To reduce the alcoholic content, pour the herbal spirits into a cup, add 30–60 ml of boiling water, and let sit for a few minutes so that some of the alcohol evaporates. The best times to drink herbal spirits are just before dinner and shortly before bedtime, but in cold winter weather the first dose may be taken at midday to help warm the body.

Tonic spirits should only be taken when you're feeling healthy and well balanced. When ill or disordered, discontinue all tonics and switch to curative therapies until health and balance are restored.

Mail-order Suppliers

Most of the products mentioned in this book can be obtained in one form or another from health food shops in major cities and towns throughout the world, or by mail-order through various websites on the Internet. The suppliers listed below are those from whom the author has been ordering for many years. They supply top-quality products at reasonable prices, and all of them offer a worldwide mail-order service.

V. E. Irons Inc. & Colema Boards Inc.
P.O. Box 34710
North Kansas City, MO 64116 USA
tel: **1 800 544–8147, 1 816 221–3719**
fax: **1 816 221–1272**
website: **www.veirons.com and www.colema.com**
email: **info@veirons.com and info@colema.com**

The Irons family supplies the entire line of V.E. Irons' Vitratox brand of internal cleansing products, which the author highly recommends as supplements for any sort of therapeutic fasting programme. They also supply several models of the famous Colema Board for doing colonic irrigations at home, and provide detailed printed material regarding the seven-day internal cleansing fast and colonic irrigation programme developed by

V. E Irons. The Irons programme is the fastest and most effective way to conduct complete detox and internal organ cleansing programmes at home.

Products: Intestinal Cleanser (psyllium powder); Detoxificant (liquid bentonite); Greenlife (cereal grass juice tablets); Enzymatic Supplement (digestive enzymes); Herb Tablets (herbal laxative); Colema Board (colonic irrigation kit); and additional related items.

Dragon River Herbals
P.O. Box 28
El Rito, NM 87530 USA
tel: **1 505 583–2348**
fax: **1 505 583–2339**
website: **www.dragonriverherbals.com**
email: **info@dragonriverherbals.com**

Dragon River Herbals produces a wide range of high-potency liquid extracts and herbal tinctures from top-grade medicinal herbs, including traditional Western as well as Chinese varieties. In addition to dozens of single-herb tinctures, Dragon River also blends a line of its own herbal formulas specially designed for specific conditions by master herbalist Charlie Jordon. As pure concentrated extracts, these formulas produce swift therapeutic results and are very convenient to use at home, at work or while travelling. For information and instructions regarding the use of these herbal remedies, you may order a copy of Charlie Jordon's *Restorative Herbal Guidebook* from Dragon River.

Products: Single herb extracts, including those required for a parasite programme (black walnut hull, wormwood, clove); Rejuvenate (liver detox formula); Life Support (immune enhancer); Lights Out (nervine relaxant for sleep); Breath of Life (lung and respiratory remedy); Peace & Quiet (anti-hypertensive relaxant); and many others.

Fruitful Yield
P.O. Box 6247
Bloomingdale, IL 60108–6247 USA
tel: 1 800 469–5552, 1 630 351-9156
fax: 1 630 351–9430
website: www.FruitfulYieldDirect.com
email: sales@FruitfulYieldDirect.com

This company supplies the complete line of NOW brand vitamins, minerals and other nutritional supplements, as well as herbal extracts, 'green foods', essential oils and other health products. NOW supplements are among the purest on the market today, produced only with natural ingredients without the use of chemical additives, and new products based on the latest discoveries in naturopathic health research are added to their line regularly.
Products: Alkaline vitamin C; vitamin E with selenium; beta-carotene; multi-vitamin and mineral formulas; spirulina; chlorella; calcium citrate with magnesium; stevia powder or extract (natural herbal sweetener); lactobacteria supplements; digestive enzymes; antioxidant formulas; sage, lavender, rosemary, peppermint, and other essential oils; and related health products.

Sandent Co.
514 Greenland Drive
Murfreesboro, TN 37130 USA
tel: 1 615 890–9832
website: www.sandent.com

Sandent is the USA supplier for the ESF energized water supplement, which releases free oxygen and hydrogen into the bloodstream. This product is also known as Liquid Life and Cell Food, depending on where it's being sold. For more details on this product, and the names of suppliers in other parts of the world, check the manufacturer's website: nuscience.com
Product: ESF/Cell Food/Liquid Life.

Inner Glow Health Products
P.O. Box 162
Tewantin, QLD 4565 Australia
tel: 61 7 5449–0600
fax: 61 7 5449-0900
email: innerglo@smart.net.au

Inner Glow supplies a broad selection of health products for self-health care at home, including nutritional and herbal supplements, natural body care products, and a variety of high-tech electro-detox devices. Their line of products expands continuously and includes many items that are difficult to find elsewhere. Printed copies of clinical studies and other scientific research regarding their products is available on request.
Products: Herbal Fibre Blend (psyllium with cleansing herbs); Mag-i-Cal (ionized magnesium and calcium supplement); Triplex Formula (for parasites); Grander Water System; Barley Green; Dead Sea Bath Salts; Dead Sea Mud (for skin detox); ESF Liquid Life, BEFE (bio-electric field enhancer); Zapper (electro-parasite device); ionizers; and many other products for internal and external health care.

Acuneeds
622 Camberwell Road
Camberwell, VIC 3124 Australia
tel: 1 800 678–789, 61 3 9889–4100
fax: 61 3 9889-1200
website: www.acuneeds.com
email: info@acuneeds.com

Acuneeds supplies traditional Chinese herbal formulas, as well as single herbs, produced by the most reputable herbal medicine makers in China and Taiwan. Available as tablets, powders, freeze-dried granules, teas, ointments and creams these remedies are convenient and economical to use for prolonged periods of herbal

therapy at home. Acuneeds also supplies acupuncture needles, moxibustion and other TCM supplies, and offers a variety of books for sale on various aspects of Chinese herbal medicine.
Products: Traditional Chinese herbal formulas and single herbs.

Ion Life
Byron Bay, Australia
tel: **61 2 66856471, 61 2 66856473**
fax: **61 2 66856473**
website: **www.ionlife.info**
email: **info@ionlife.info**

Ion Life specializes in supplying various types of home ionizers for both air and water, including water ionizers for making micro-clustered alkaline water and the GEOMED negative ion generator for concentrated negative ion breathing therapy.
Products: Drinking water purifiers and ionizers; GEOMED negative ion air generator.

Siamese Traders
85, Sukaseam Rd, Soi 12
T-Patan, A. Muang
Chiang Mai 50300 Thailand
tel: **66 53 409705, 66 53 409171**
fax: **66 53 409113**
email: **nikolaus@siamesetraders.com**

Siamese Traders supplies a variety of high-quality health products organically produced in northern Thailand, including natural health foods and herbal teas, herbal body care products, Celtic-style sea salts and High Mountain Oolung Tea grown in Thailand from plants brought there from the highlands of Taiwan. All products are attractively packaged and reasonably priced, and many of them may be used to support the various detox programmes and daily dietary guidelines introduced in this book.

Products: Whole sea salt (plain or blended with chilli and other Thai herbs); herbal teas; Cooling Herbal Body Powder; Healing Herbal Skin Balm; traditional Thai herbal steam formulas; High Mountain Oolung Tea and other Chinese teas; Bliss Bio-Circuit (silk energy balancer); tea leaf pillows; and many other fine products.

The Centre for Implosion Research
P.O. Box 38
Plymouth PL7 5YX, UK
tel: **01752 345552**
fax: **01752 338569**
website: **www.ImplosionResearch.com**
email: **enquiries@ImplosionResearch.com**

The Centre for Implosion Research is involved in subtle energy and water research and manufactures a range of products that are despatched all over the world.
Product: Vortex Energizer

OTT-LITE Technology
1214 West Cass Street
Tampa, FL 33606 USA
tel: **813 621 0058**
fax: **813 626 8790**
website: **www.ott-lite.com**

These are suppliers of a range of speciality environmental lighting concepts.
Product: Ott-Lite

The Grain & Salt Society
273 Fairway Drive
Asheville, NC 28805 USA
tel: **704 299 9005**
fax: **704 299 1640**
website: **www.celtic-seasalt.com**

This company is an excellent source of the best grade Celtic Seas Salt from Brittany, as well as other related products.
Product: Celtic Sea Salt

EPRT Technologies, Inc.
P.O. Box 278
Pacific Palisades, CA 90272 USA
tel: **888 838 4008**
fax: **310 459 0195**

This company produces and distributes the most amazing Jai machine, mentioned in the Electro-Detox chapter.
Product: Jai machine

Herbal Suppliers in the UK

Acumedic Ltd.
101–105 Camden High Street
London NW1 7JN
tel: 020 73886704

East West Natural Health
Langston Priory Mews
Kingham
Oxfordshire OX7 6UP
tel: 01608 658862

Retail Shop and Clinic
3 Neals Yard
London WC2H 9DP
tel: 020 73791312

The following organisations may be useful for more information on suppliers and practitioners in the UK.

British Acupuncture Council (BAC)
tel: 020 87350400
website: www.acupuncture.org.uk

Register of Chinese Herbal Medicine
Office 5, Ferndale Business Centre
1 Exeter Street
Norwich NR2 4QB
tel: 01603 623994
fax: 01603 467557
email: herbmed@rchm.co.uk
website: www.rchm.co.uk

Index

(page numbers in *italic type* refer to illustrations)

POCKET
BOOKS

THE TAO OF HEALTH, SEX AND LONGEVITY

A Modern Practical Approach to the Ancient Way

Daniel Reid

People are incresingly looking to alternatives to
Western medicine and here is a practical self-help
guide to a balanced and positive lifestyle.

Tao, the most ancient and fundamental element in
the world's oldest civilization, is as relevant to
today's world as to classical China. For the contemporary reader, this accessible book is the first to
explore, in the light of the findings of Western
science, the balanced and holistic system of health
care used by Chinese physcians, martial artists and
meditators for over 5,000 years.

ISBN 0 7434 0907 8
PRICE £8.99

POCKET
BOOKS

GUARDING THE THREE TREASURES
The Chinese Way of Health

Daniel Reid

A companion volume to THE TAO OF HEALTH,
SEX AND LONGEVITY, this is an indispensable
introduction to the philosophy and practice of
Taoist health care.

The way of Tao is the way of harmony with nature,
a dynamic balance of Yin and Yang. Maintaining
this balance in your own mind and body will
strengthen your immune system and build up your
general health. Whereas western medicine attempts
to fix the affected body part or organ when something goes wrong, Chinese medicine takes a
holisitic and preventative approach and let you take
charge, through diet and exercises, of your mental
and physical well being.

ISBN 0 7434 0906 X
PRICE £8.99